ATRIAL FIBRILLATION

UNVEILING THE CAUSES, PREVENTION AND TREATMENT OPTIONS

Dr. Givens Bestman

DISCLAIMER

Copyright © Dr. Givens Bestman 2023. All Rights Reserved.

Table of Contents

INTRODUCTION

Atrial fibrillation is a common cardiac arrhythmia characterized by an irregular and rapid heartbeat. Understanding the causes, prevention, and treatment options for this condition is crucial for both healthcare professionals and individuals affected by atrial fibrillation. This comprehensive guide aims to provide valuable insights into the intricacies of atrial fibrillation, its underlying causes, effective preventive measures, and various treatment options available. By delving into the anatomy, pathophysiology, and risk factors associated with atrial fibrillation, as well as the potential complications it poses, this resource equips readers with the knowledge necessary to navigate this complex condition. Moreover, it emphasizes the importance of timely diagnosis, lifestyle modifications, and appropriate medical interventions to effectively manage atrial fibrillation and enhance overall well-being.

Overview of Atrial Fibrillation

This section provides a comprehensive overview of atrial fibrillation, including its definition, types, and underlying mechanisms. It explores the impact of AF on the heart's function and discusses the potential symptoms that individuals may experience. Understanding the nature and manifestations of atrial fibrillation is crucial for accurate diagnosis and effective management.

Importance of Understanding the Causes, Prevention, and Treatment Options

Understanding the causes of atrial fibrillation is vital in addressing the root factors that contribute to its development. By identifying and managing underlying conditions like hypertension, heart diseases, and thyroid disorders, healthcare professionals can help mitigate the risk of AF and its complications.

Furthermore, knowledge of prevention strategies empowers individuals to make lifestyle modifications that can reduce the likelihood of developing atrial fibrillation. By adopting healthy habits, managing weight, controlling blood pressure, and limiting alcohol intake, individuals can actively protect their heart health.

Lastly, being aware of the available treatment options for atrial fibrillation enables individuals and healthcare providers to make informed decisions about the most appropriate interventions. This includes medication therapies, electrical cardioversion, ablation procedures, or surgical interventions. Tailoring the treatment plan based on individual needs can improve symptom management, reduce the risk of complications, and enhance overall quality of life.

In conclusion, a thorough understanding of atrial fibrillation's overview, including its causes, prevention strategies, and treatment options, is crucial for effective management and improved patient outcomes.

By equipping individuals with this knowledge, they can actively participate in their healthcare, make informed decisions, and take proactive steps to minimize the impact of atrial fibrillation on their lives.

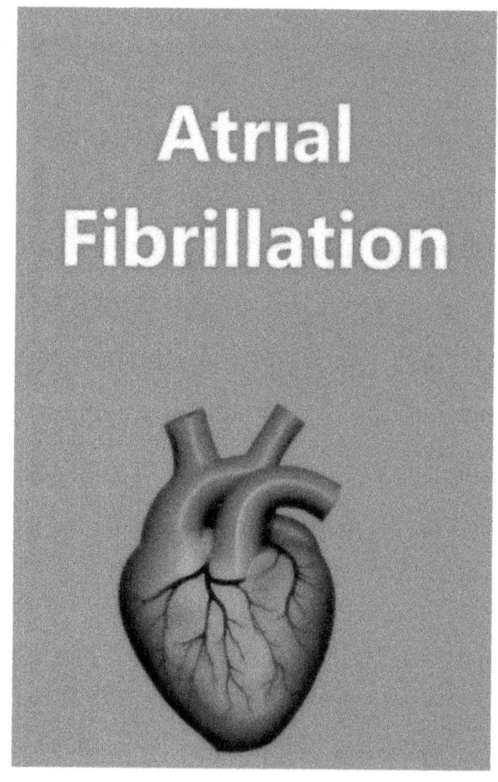

CHAPTER ONE

Understanding Atrial Fibrillation

Millions of people worldwide are afflicted by atrial fibrillation (AF), a common heart arrhythmia. It is characterized by irregular and often rapid electrical impulses in the atria, the upper chambers of the heart. This irregularity disrupts the normal rhythm of the heart and can have significant implications for cardiovascular health.

To understand atrial fibrillation, it is important to grasp the underlying mechanisms and causes. AF occurs when the electrical signals in the atria become chaotic, causing the atria to quiver or fibrillate instead of contracting in a coordinated manner. This irregular electrical activity can be influenced by a variety of factors, including age, genetics, heart disease, high blood pressure, obesity, thyroid disorders, and other medical conditions. The impact of atrial fibrillation on the body can be far-reaching.

The irregular and ineffective pumping of blood from the atria can lead to decreased blood flow to the rest of the body, potentially causing symptoms such as palpitations, shortness of breath, fatigue, dizziness, and chest discomfort. AF also carries an increased risk of complications, most notably blood clot formation in the atria. If a blood clot dislodges and travels to the brain, it can cause a stroke, making stroke prevention a crucial aspect of managing AF.

Diagnosing atrial fibrillation involves a comprehensive evaluation that may include a thorough medical history, physical examination, and various diagnostic tests. Electrocardiogram (ECG) is commonly used to identify the characteristic irregular heartbeat pattern of AF. Other tests such as Holter monitoring, echocardiography, and blood tests may be employed to assess underlying causes, evaluate heart function, and identify any associated conditions or complications.

Managing atrial fibrillation requires a multi-faceted approach tailored to each individual's specific circumstances. Treatment goals typically include restoring and maintaining a normal heart rhythm, controlling heart rate, reducing the risk of blood clots, and managing underlying conditions that may contribute to AF. Treatment options may include medications to regulate heart rhythm and rate, anticoagulant therapy to prevent blood clots, lifestyle modifications (e.g., managing stress, maintaining a healthy weight, avoiding triggers), and, techniques like cardioversion or catheter ablation in specific circumstances.

Regular monitoring and follow-up care are essential for individuals with atrial fibrillation. This helps healthcare providers assess treatment effectiveness, adjust medications as needed, monitor for complications, and ensure overall cardiovascular health. It is important for patients to actively participate in their care, adhere to prescribed treatments, and engage in lifestyle modifications to manage their condition effectively.

Understanding atrial fibrillation empowers individuals to make informed decisions about their health and take steps to prevent complications. By working closely with healthcare providers, staying educated about the condition, and adopting a heart-healthy lifestyle, individuals with atrial fibrillation can optimize their well-being, reduce symptoms, and minimize the risk of stroke and other cardiovascular complications associated with AF.

Definition of Atrial Fibrillation

Rapid and erratic electrical impulses in the heart's atria are the hallmarks of atrial fibrillation (AF), a frequent cardiac arrhythmia. In a healthy heart, electrical signals coordinate the contraction of the atria and ventricles, ensuring an efficient blood pumping process. However, in atrial fibrillation, this normal rhythm is disrupted, leading to chaotic and disorganized electrical activity.

The atria do not efficiently contract during atrial fibrillation. Instead, they quiver or fibrillate, resulting in an irregular heartbeat. This irregularity can manifest as a rapid, irregular, or fluttering pulse.

The atria's ineffective contractions may cause blood to pool or stagnate, increasing the risk of blood clot formation.

Atrial fibrillation can occur in episodes, with the heart spontaneously returning to a normal rhythm (paroxysmal AF), or it can persist and require intervention to restore a normal rhythm (persistent AF). In some cases, atrial fibrillation may become a permanent condition (permanent AF) that cannot be reversed, even with medical intervention.

AF is often associated with other underlying heart conditions, such as hypertension (high blood pressure), coronary artery disease, heart failure, or heart valve problems. However, it can also occur without any apparent underlying heart disease, known as nonvalvular atrial fibrillation.

The irregular electrical activity of AF disrupts the heart's pumping efficiency, potentially affecting blood flow to the rest of the body.

As a result, individuals with atrial fibrillation may experience various symptoms, including palpitations, shortness of breath, fatigue, dizziness, chest discomfort, or even fainting. However, it's important to note that some individuals may be asymptomatic, and atrial fibrillation may only be detected during routine medical check-ups or diagnostic tests.

The consequences of atrial fibrillation extend beyond its immediate symptoms. It significantly increases the risk of complications, including stroke, heart failure, and other heart-related issues. The irregular blood flow in the atria can cause blood clots to form, which can then travel to the brain, leading to a stroke. Therefore, stroke prevention strategies, such as anticoagulation therapy, are an essential component of managing atrial fibrillation.

Accurate diagnosis and classification of atrial fibrillation are crucial for determining the most appropriate treatment strategies.

Treatment goals for AF include restoring and maintaining a normal heart rhythm, controlling heart rate, preventing blood clot formation, and managing underlying conditions contributing to AF.

In summary, atrial fibrillation is a cardiac arrhythmia characterized by irregular and rapid electrical impulses in the atria of the heart. It can manifest as episodes or persist continuously and is associated with various symptoms and potential complications. Accurate diagnosis and understanding of atrial fibrillation are fundamental for appropriate management and the prevention of associated risks.

Classification of Atrial Fibrillation

Atrial fibrillation (AF) can be classified based on several factors, including the duration, persistence, and underlying causes or contributing factors.

Understanding the different classifications of AF is crucial for accurate diagnosis, treatment selection, and predicting the prognosis of the condition.

Duration-Based Classification:

a) Paroxysmal Atrial Fibrillation (PAF):

Paroxysmal AF refers to episodes of atrial fibrillation that start suddenly and resolve spontaneously within 7 days, typically within 48 hours. The episodes may last for seconds, minutes, hours, or up to 7 days before returning to a normal heart rhythm. Individuals with PAF often experience intermittent episodes of atrial fibrillation, followed by periods of normal heart rhythm. These episodes may occur spontaneously or be triggered by specific factors, such as stress, exercise, or caffeine intake.

b) Persistent Atrial Fibrillation:

Persistent AF occurs when the abnormal heart rhythm lasts for more than 7 days and requires intervention to restore a normal rhythm. Unlike paroxysmal AF, persistent AF does not spontaneously convert to a normal rhythm.

Medical intervention, such as electrical cardioversion or medication, is typically needed to restore a normal heart rhythm. Persistent AF can last for an extended period, with episodes lasting weeks, months, or even years.

c) Long-standing Persistent Atrial Fibrillation:

Long-standing persistent AF refers to continuous AF lasting for more than 12 months. In this classification, attempts to restore a normal heart rhythm have been unsuccessful, and the condition becomes chronic. Long-standing persistent AF may require a combination of treatment approaches, including medications and procedures, to manage the symptoms and improve the patient's quality of life.

d) Permanent Atrial Fibrillation:

Permanent AF occurs when attempts to restore a normal heart rhythm have been intentionally stopped or have been unsuccessful. In this classification, the irregular heart rhythm becomes a persistent and long-term condition.

The focus of treatment shifts towards managing symptoms, controlling heart rate, and preventing complications rather than attempting to restore a normal rhythm.

Cause-based Classification:

a) Nonvalvular Atrial Fibrillation:

Nonvalvular AF refers to atrial fibrillation that occurs in the absence of significant heart valve disease as the underlying cause. Most cases of atrial fibrillation fall under this category. Nonvalvular AF is typically associated with risk factors such as age, hypertension, obesity, diabetes, and underlying heart conditions like coronary artery disease or heart failure.

b) Valvular Atrial Fibrillation:

Valvular AF occurs when atrial fibrillation is associated with significant heart valve disease, such as mitral valve stenosis or mitral valve regurgitation. Valve-related issues can disrupt the normal flow of blood through the heart and contribute to the development of atrial fibrillation. Valvular AF may require specific considerations in treatment, including the management of the underlying valve disease.

Understanding the classification of atrial fibrillation helps healthcare professionals determine the appropriate treatment approach for each individual. It enables personalized management strategies that address the specific type of AF, its underlying causes, and associated risk factors. Treatment goals focus on restoring and maintaining a normal heart rhythm, controlling heart rate, preventing complications, and optimizing the patient's overall cardiovascular health.

Anatomy and Physiology of the Heart in Relation to Atrial Fibrillation

To understand the impact of atrial fibrillation (AF) on the heart, it is important to have a solid understanding of the anatomy and physiology of this vital organ. The heart is a complex muscular organ located in the chest, responsible for pumping oxygenated blood to the body's tissues and organs. Let's explore the anatomy and physiology of the heart in relation to AF:

Anatomy of the Heart:

Two upper chambers, known as atria (plural: atrium), and two lower chambers, known as ventricles, make up the four chambers of the heart. Via the superior and inferior vena cava, the right atrium gets blood that has lost oxygen (deoxygenated). It then contracts, forcing the blood into the right ventricle. The right ventricle pumps this deoxygenated blood into the lungs for oxygenation through the pulmonary artery.

Via the pulmonary veins, oxygenated blood travels from the lungs back to the left atrium. The left atrium contracts, propelling the blood into the left ventricle. The left ventricle, which is the heart's main pumping chamber, contracts forcefully, pumping the oxygenated blood to the rest of the body through the aorta.

The mitral valve, also referred to as the bicuspid valve, separates the left atrium from the left ventricle, whereas the tricuspid valve separates the right atrium from the right ventricle.

As opposed to the aortic valve, which separates the left ventricle from the aorta, the pulmonary valve is located between the right ventricle and the pulmonary artery.

Physiology of the Heart:

The heart's beating or cardiac cycle is a precisely coordinated sequence of events driven by electrical impulses that regulate its contractions. Normally, these electrical signals originate from a specialized cluster of cells in the right atrium called the sinoatrial (SA) node, often referred to as the heart's natural pacemaker. The SA node generates electrical impulses that spread across the atria, causing them to contract and push blood into the ventricles.

The electrical impulses then travel through the atrioventricular (AV) node, located between the atria and ventricles.

The AV node delays the signals for a brief moment, allowing the atria to contract fully before the impulses reach the ventricles. From the AV node, the impulses are conducted through specialized pathways called the bundle of His and its branches, which deliver the signals to the ventricles. This coordinated electrical activity ensures efficient pumping of blood by the heart.

In the case of atrial fibrillation, the electrical signals within the atria become chaotic and disorganized. Instead of the normal coordinated contractions, the atria fibrillate or quiver, resulting in ineffective pumping of blood into the ventricles. The irregular electrical activity overrides the normal electrical impulses from the SA node, leading to the loss of the atrial kick, which is the contribution of atrial contraction to ventricular filling.

The irregular and rapid electrical activity in the atria during AF can cause the ventricles to beat irregularly as well, leading to an irregular heart rate. The irregular heart rhythm and reduced efficiency of pumping can result in symptoms such as palpitations, fatigue, and shortness of breath.

Understanding the anatomy and physiology of the heart in relation to AF provides valuable insights into the impact of this arrhythmia on the heart's function. It highlights how the disruption of normal electrical activity in the atria can result in irregular contractions, affecting the heart's ability to pump blood effectively. By recognizing these physiological changes, healthcare providers can develop appropriate treatment strategies to manage AF and minimize its impact on overall cardiac function.

It is important to consult with a healthcare professional for a comprehensive evaluation and personalized management plan if you suspect or have been diagnosed with atrial fibrillation. A thorough understanding of the anatomy and physiology of the heart aids in the appreciation of the complexities of AF and facilitates informed discussions between patients and healthcare providers regarding treatment options and long-term management strategies.

Pathophysiology of Atrial Fibrillation

Atrial fibrillation (AF) is a complex arrhythmia with a multifactorial pathophysiology involving electrical, structural, and functional changes in the heart. Understanding the underlying mechanisms of AF can shed light on its development, progression, and potential treatment strategies. Here, we delve into the pathophysiology of atrial fibrillation in detail.

Electrical Remodeling:

AF typically starts with the initiation of ectopic electrical impulses originating from the pulmonary veins or other atrial regions. These impulses disrupt the normal conduction of electrical signals within the atria. In atrial fibrillation, the atrial tissue undergoes electrical remodeling, which involves alterations in ion channel expression and electrical properties of cardiomyocytes.

This remodeling enhances the susceptibility of atrial tissue to abnormal electrical activity, making it more prone to reentry and fibrillation.

Triggers and Reentry:

A common trigger for atrial fibrillation is rapid and irregular firing of ectopic beats originating from the pulmonary veins. These triggers can initiate reentry circuits within the atria. Reentry occurs when a wave of electrical activity circulates within the atrial tissue, causing sustained and disorganized electrical impulses. The reentrant circuits can be localized or widespread, leading to the chaotic atrial electrical activity observed in AF.

Structural Changes:

Structural changes in the atria play a significant role in the development and perpetuation of AF. Conditions such as atrial dilation, fibrosis (abnormal deposition of collagen), and atrial myopathy (structural abnormalities in the atrial tissue) can promote the initiation and maintenance of AF. Structural remodeling alters the electrical properties of the atrial tissue, creating a substrate that supports the perpetuation of abnormal electrical activity.

Autonomic Nervous System Influence:

The autonomic nervous system, specifically the sympathetic and parasympathetic branches, can modulate the occurrence and severity of atrial fibrillation. Increased sympathetic activity and decreased parasympathetic (vagal) tone have been associated with atrial fibrillation. The autonomic nervous system's influence on atrial electrophysiology can promote electrical instability, trigger ectopic beats, and contribute to the progression of AF.

Atrial Thrombogenesis:

Atrial fibrillation disrupts the coordinated contraction of the atria, leading to stagnant blood flow and the formation of blood clots (thrombi) in the atria. These blood clots can embolize, causing strokes or other systemic thromboembolic events.

The risk of thromboembolism is particularly high in individuals with additional risk factors such as underlying heart disease, age, hypertension, diabetes, or prior history of stroke.

Additional Factors:

Other factors, such as inflammation, oxidative stress, genetic predisposition, and metabolic disturbances, have also been implicated in the pathophysiology of atrial fibrillation. These factors can contribute to the underlying substrate for AF by further promoting electrical and structural remodeling within the atria.

In summary, the pathophysiology of atrial fibrillation involves a complex interplay of electrical, structural, and functional changes in the atrial tissue. Electrical remodeling, triggers, reentry, structural alterations, autonomic nervous system influence, and the risk of thromboembolism all contribute to the development and progression of atrial fibrillation.

Understanding these underlying mechanisms is essential for developing targeted treatment strategies aimed at restoring and maintaining a normal heart rhythm, preventing complications, and improving the overall management of atrial fibrillation.

CHAPTER TWO

Causes and Risk Factors of Atrial Fibrillation

Atrial fibrillation (AF) can develop as a result of various causes and is influenced by several risk factors. Understanding these underlying factors is essential in diagnosing and managing this common cardiac arrhythmia. Let's delve into the causes and risk factors associated with AF:

Causes of Atrial Fibrillation:

1. Age:

Advancing age is a significant risk factor for AF, with the prevalence increasing with each decade of life. The structural and electrical changes that occur in the heart over time can contribute to the development of AF.

2. Heart Diseases:

Various heart conditions can trigger or exacerbate AF. These include coronary artery disease, heart failure, valve disorders (such as mitral valve disease), congenital heart defects, and cardiomyopathies.

The presence of these underlying heart diseases disrupts the normal electrical activity in the atria, increasing the likelihood of AF.

3. High Blood Pressure:

Hypertension (high blood pressure) is a well-established risk factor for AF. Elevated blood pressure causes structural changes in the heart, promoting electrical instability and favoring the occurrence of AF.

4. Hyperthyroidism:

Overactive thyroid gland (hyperthyroidism) can increase the risk of developing AF. Excess thyroid hormones can disrupt the normal electrical signaling in the heart, leading to arrhythmias like AF.

5. Obstructive Sleep Apnea:

Sleep apnea, a condition characterized by interrupted breathing during sleep, is associated with an increased risk of AF. The intermittent oxygen deprivation and physiological stress imposed by sleep apnea can contribute to the development and progression of AF.

Risk Factors for Atrial Fibrillation:

1. Family History:

There is a genetic component to AF, and individuals with a family history of the condition are at higher risk. A person's susceptibility to irregular cardiac rhythms, such as AF, might be predisposed by specific genetic abnormalities.

2. Lifestyle Factors:

Unhealthy lifestyle choices can contribute to the development of AF. They include binge drinking, smoking, being overweight, not exercising, and eating poorly. Addressing these modifiable risk factors can help reduce the risk of AF and its complications.

3. Chronic Conditions:

Several chronic conditions are associated with an increased risk of AF. These include diabetes, chronic kidney disease, lung disease, and metabolic syndrome. Proper management of these conditions is crucial in reducing the risk of AF.

4. Previous Cardiac Procedures:

Individuals who have undergone cardiac surgeries, such as open-heart surgery or valve replacements may have an increased risk of developing AF. This is due to the disruption of normal heart tissue and electrical pathways during these procedures.

5. Other Factors:

Certain medical conditions and lifestyle factors can contribute to AF. These include excessive caffeine or stimulant intake, excessive stress or anxiety, use of certain medications or substances (e.g., stimulant drugs), and electrolyte imbalances.

While these causes and risk factors are associated with an increased likelihood of developing AF, it's important to note that AF can also occur without any identifiable cause or in individuals without any known risk factors. It highlights the complex nature of AF and the need for individualized assessment and management.

By understanding the causes and risk factors of AF, healthcare providers can better identify individuals at risk, initiate appropriate diagnostic evaluations, and implement strategies to prevent or manage AF effectively. For individuals, awareness of these factors can help promote heart-healthy habits, encourage regular medical check-ups, and facilitate early intervention when necessary.

Common Causes of Atrial Fibrillation

Atrial fibrillation (AF) can have various underlying causes and contributing factors.

Identifying these causes is crucial for understanding the risk factors, implementing preventive measures, and managing the condition effectively. Here are some of the common causes of atrial fibrillation:

Age:

Age is a significant risk factor for atrial fibrillation, with the prevalence of AF increasing with advancing age. The exact mechanisms underlying the age-related increase in AF risk are not fully understood, but factors such as structural changes in the atria, fibrosis, and electrical remodeling may play a role.

Hypertension:

Hypertension, or high blood pressure, is closely linked to the development of atrial fibrillation. Elevated blood pressure can cause structural changes in the heart, such as left ventricular hypertrophy, which can disrupt the normal electrical conduction in the atria and promote the onset of AF.

Coronary Artery Disease:

Coronary artery disease (CAD) occurs when the blood vessels supplying the heart muscle become narrowed or blocked due to atherosclerosis. CAD can lead to inadequate blood flow and oxygen supply to the heart, increasing the risk of atrial fibrillation. Ischemia or damage to the atrial tissue caused by reduced blood flow can disrupt the normal electrical pathways.

Structural Heart Disease:

Various structural abnormalities or heart diseases can contribute to the development of atrial fibrillation. These include:

- **Valvular Heart Disease:** Conditions such as mitral valve disease, especially mitral valve stenosis or regurgitation, can disrupt the normal flow of blood through the heart and contribute to the development of atrial fibrillation.

- **Cardiomyopathy:** Dilated cardiomyopathy, hypertrophic cardiomyopathy, or other types of cardiomyopathies can lead to atrial enlargement, fibrosis, and electrical remodeling, increasing the risk of AF.

- **Congenital Heart Defects:** Certain congenital heart abnormalities, such as atrial septal defects or atrial myxomas, can create a substrate for atrial fibrillation.

Thyroid Disorders:

Thyroid disorders, particularly hyperthyroidism (overactive thyroid), can increase the risk of atrial fibrillation. The excessive production of thyroid hormones can disrupt normal cardiac function, leading to arrhythmias, including AF.

Obesity and Metabolic Syndrome:

Obesity and metabolic syndrome, characterized by a combination of obesity, high blood pressure, abnormal blood sugar levels, and abnormal lipid profile, are associated with an increased risk of atrial fibrillation. These conditions contribute to the development of structural and electrical changes in the heart, promoting AF.

Sleep Apnea:

Sleep apnea, a disorder characterized by repeated pauses in breathing during sleep, has been linked to atrial fibrillation. The intermittent hypoxia and increased sympathetic activity associated with sleep apnea can trigger abnormal electrical activity in the atria, promoting AF.

Other Factors:

Several other factors can increase the risk of atrial fibrillation, including excessive alcohol consumption, stimulant use (such as cocaine or amphetamines), chronic kidney disease, lung disease, and a family history of AF. Genetic factors may also play a role in predisposing individuals to AF.

It's important to note that in some cases, the cause of atrial fibrillation may be unknown, particularly in nonvalvular AF. Identifying the underlying cause or contributing factors of AF is essential for guiding treatment decisions, implementing preventive measures, and managing the overall cardiovascular health of individuals with AF.

Underlying Medical Conditions Associated with Atrial Fibrillation

Atrial fibrillation (AF) is often associated with underlying medical conditions that contribute to its development and progression. Understanding these associated conditions is vital for accurate diagnosis, risk assessment, and comprehensive management of AF. Here are some of the common underlying medical conditions associated with atrial fibrillation:

Hypertension:

High blood pressure, also known as hypertension, poses a serious risk for atrial fibrillation. Prolonged elevation of blood pressure can lead to structural changes in the heart, such as left ventricular hypertrophy, atrial enlargement, and fibrosis. These alterations disrupt the normal electrical conduction in the atria, increasing the risk of AF development.

Coronary Artery Disease:

Coronary artery disease (CAD), characterized by the narrowing or blockage of coronary arteries, is associated with an increased risk of atrial fibrillation.

Reduced blood flow to the heart muscle due to CAD can lead to ischemia or damage in the atrial tissue, promoting the development of arrhythmias like AF.

Structural Heart Disease:

Various structural abnormalities or heart diseases can contribute to the occurrence of atrial fibrillation. These include:

- **Valvular Heart Disease:** Conditions such as mitral valve disease, especially mitral valve stenosis or regurgitation, can disrupt the normal flow of blood through the heart, increasing the risk of atrial fibrillation.

- **Cardiomyopathy:** Different types of cardiomyopathy, including dilated cardiomyopathy, hypertrophic cardiomyopathy, and restrictive cardiomyopathy, can lead to atrial enlargement, fibrosis, and electrical remodeling, predisposing individuals to AF.

- **Congenital Heart Defects:** Certain congenital heart abnormalities, such as atrial septal defects or atrial myxomas, can create a substrate for atrial fibrillation.

Heart Failure:

Heart failure, a condition characterized by the heart's inability to pump blood effectively, is strongly associated with atrial fibrillation.

The structural and functional changes in the heart that occur in heart failure, such as atrial dilation, fibrosis, and impaired contractility, significantly increase the risk of developing AF.

Thyroid Disorders:

Thyroid disorders, particularly hyperthyroidism (overactive thyroid) and to a lesser extent hypothyroidism (underactive thyroid), are known to be associated with atrial fibrillation. The excessive production or insufficient levels of thyroid hormones can disrupt normal cardiac function and electrical conduction, leading to arrhythmias like AF.

Chronic Kidney Disease:

Chronic kidney disease (CKD), a condition characterized by the gradual loss of kidney function, has been identified as a risk factor for atrial fibrillation. The precise mechanisms linking CKD to AF are not fully understood, but factors such as electrolyte imbalances, inflammation, and uremic toxins may contribute to the increased risk.

Obstructive Sleep Apnea:

Obstructive sleep apnea, a sleep disorder characterized by recurrent pauses in breathing during sleep, is closely associated with atrial fibrillation. The intermittent hypoxia, increased sympathetic activity, and intrathoracic pressure changes associated with sleep apnea can trigger abnormal electrical activity in the atria, promoting AF.

Other Conditions:

Several other medical conditions have been linked to an increased risk of atrial fibrillation, including diabetes mellitus, chronic obstructive pulmonary disease (COPD), obesity, hyperthyroidism, and a history of prior stroke or transient ischemic attack (TIA). Additionally, a family history of AF and certain genetic factors may predispose individuals to develop atrial fibrillation.

Identifying and managing underlying medical conditions associated with atrial fibrillation is crucial for effective management of the arrhythmia.

A comprehensive approach that addresses these conditions through lifestyle modifications, medication management, and appropriate interventions can help reduce the risk of AF recurrence, complications, and improve overall cardiovascular health.

Lifestyle Factors and Environmental Influences

In addition to underlying medical conditions, lifestyle factors and environmental influences can significantly impact the development, progression, and management of atrial fibrillation (AF). Modifying these factors can play a vital role in reducing the risk of AF and improving overall heart health. Here are some important lifestyle factors and environmental influences associated with atrial fibrillation:

Alcohol Consumption:

Excessive alcohol consumption has been identified as a risk factor for atrial fibrillation. Alcohol can disrupt the electrical signaling in the heart, leading to arrhythmias.

Additionally, alcohol can increase blood pressure and trigger other cardiac events, which can contribute to the onset of AF. Limiting alcohol intake or avoiding it altogether is recommended, especially for individuals with a history of AF or at risk for developing the condition.

Smoking:

Smoking tobacco products, including cigarettes and cigars, has been strongly linked to an increased risk of atrial fibrillation. The harmful chemicals in tobacco smoke can damage the heart and blood vessels, promoting inflammation, oxidative stress, and atherosclerosis. These factors can contribute to the development and progression of AF. Quitting smoking is crucial for reducing the risk of AF and improving overall cardiovascular health.

Obesity and Sedentary Lifestyle:

Obesity and a sedentary lifestyle are associated with a higher risk of atrial fibrillation. Excess body weight and a lack of physical activity can contribute to hypertension, diabetes, dyslipidemia, and structural changes in the heart, all of which increase the likelihood of AF development.

Maintaining a healthy weight through a balanced diet and regular exercise can help reduce the risk of AF and improve overall cardiovascular fitness.

Physical Activity:

Regular physical activity is beneficial for cardiovascular health and can help reduce the risk of atrial fibrillation. Engaging in moderate-intensity aerobic exercises, such as brisk walking, swimming, or cycling, for at least 150 minutes per week can improve heart function, lower blood pressure, and promote overall well-being. However, intense and prolonged endurance exercises, particularly in individuals who are not accustomed to them, may increase the risk of AF in some cases. It is essential to strike a balance between exercise and individual fitness levels.

Stress and Emotional Well-being:

Chronic stress and emotional factors can influence the occurrence and progression of atrial fibrillation. Stress activates the sympathetic nervous system, leading to increased heart rate and blood pressure, which can trigger AF episodes.

Additionally, anxiety, depression, and sleep disturbances have been associated with an increased risk of AF. Managing stress through relaxation techniques, regular exercise, adequate sleep, and seeking emotional support can contribute to better heart health and potentially reduce AF burden.

Environmental Factors:

Environmental influences, such as air pollution and exposure to certain chemicals or toxins, may contribute to the development or exacerbation of atrial fibrillation. Long-term exposure to air pollution, including particulate matter and pollutants, has been associated with an increased risk of AF. Occupational exposure to chemicals like solvents and heavy metals may also play a role. Minimizing exposure to environmental pollutants and maintaining a healthy indoor and outdoor environment can help mitigate these risks.

Medication and Substance Use:

Certain medications, such as certain antiarrhythmic drugs, can increase the risk of atrial fibrillation or worsen existing AF. Illicit substance use, particularly stimulants like cocaine and amphetamines, can trigger AF episodes due to their effects on the cardiovascular system. It is important to follow prescribed medication regimens and avoid substance abuse to reduce the risk of AF complications.

Addressing lifestyle factors and environmental influences associated with atrial fibrillation is crucial for prevention and management. Adopting a heart-healthy lifestyle, including a balanced diet, regular exercise, stress management techniques, and avoiding harmful substances, can significantly reduce the risk of AF and improve overall cardiovascular health. Additionally, creating a supportive environment with clean air and minimizing exposure to pollutants can contribute to a healthier heart.

CHAPTER THREE

Recognizing the Symptoms of Atrial Fibrillation

Atrial fibrillation (AF) can present with a range of symptoms, which can vary from person to person. Some individuals may experience noticeable and bothersome symptoms, while others may be completely asymptomatic and only discover their condition during routine medical examinations or screenings. Understanding and recognizing the symptoms associated with AF is important for timely diagnosis and appropriate management. These are some typical signs to be on the lookout for:

1. Palpitations: Palpitations are the most common symptom of AF. It is described as a sensation of rapid, fluttering, or irregular heartbeat. Some may describe it as a "racing" or "pounding" sensation in the chest. Palpitations may come and go or may be persistent, depending on the individual.

2. Fatigue and Weakness: Many individuals with AF report feelings of fatigue and weakness. This can be attributed to the irregular heart rhythm and reduced efficiency of the heart's pumping action, which can affect the delivery of oxygen and nutrients to the body's tissues.

3. Shortness of Breath: A sensation of breathlessness or difficulty breathing, particularly during physical exertion or even at rest, may be a symptom of AF. The irregular and rapid heart rhythm can compromise the heart's ability to adequately pump blood, leading to fluid buildup in the lungs and causing breathlessness.

4. Dizziness and Lightheadedness: Some individuals with AF may experience episodes of dizziness or lightheadedness. This can occur due to inadequate blood supply to the brain caused by the irregular heart rhythm or reduced cardiac output.

5. Chest Discomfort: Chest discomfort or chest pain may be present in some individuals with AF.

This can range from mild discomfort to more severe chest pain, similar to angina. It is important to note that chest pain can also indicate other underlying cardiac conditions, and medical attention should be sought promptly.

6. Fainting or Loss of Consciousness: In certain cases, AF can lead to fainting or syncope. This is usually due to a sudden drop in blood pressure resulting from an irregular heart rhythm. A medical expert should examine fainting episodes to ascertain the underlying reason.

It is important to remember that some individuals with AF may not experience any noticeable symptoms, especially if the irregular heart rhythm is paroxysmal (intermittent). However, even in the absence of symptoms, AF can still pose significant health risks, such as an increased risk of stroke. This underscores the importance of regular medical check-ups and screenings to identify AF early, particularly in individuals at higher risk.

If you experience any of the above symptoms or have concerns about your heart health, it is important to seek medical attention for a thorough evaluation. Your healthcare provider can perform appropriate tests, such as an electrocardiogram (ECG), to diagnose or rule out AF and develop an individualized treatment plan.

Recognizing the symptoms of AF and seeking timely medical evaluation can lead to an accurate diagnosis, appropriate management, and improved quality of life. It is crucial to be proactive in addressing any concerns and working closely with healthcare professionals to ensure optimal heart health.

Common Signs and Symptoms of Atrial Fibrillation

Atrial fibrillation (AF) can present with various signs and symptoms, which may vary in intensity and frequency among individuals. Recognizing these common manifestations is crucial for early detection, accurate diagnosis, and prompt management of AF.

Here are the typical signs and symptoms associated with atrial fibrillation:

Palpitations:

Palpitations are a common symptom experienced by individuals with atrial fibrillation. They are described as a rapid, irregular, and often pounding sensation in the chest. Palpitations may be intermittent or persistent and can range from mild discomfort to a distressing awareness of the heart's abnormal rhythm.

Irregular Heartbeat:

A notable characteristic of atrial fibrillation is an irregular heartbeat. Instead of the normal, regular rhythm, the heart's electrical signals become chaotic, resulting in an irregular pulse. This irregularity can be detected by checking the radial pulse at the wrist or by an electrocardiogram (ECG).

Fatigue and Weakness:

Many individuals with atrial fibrillation experience fatigue and generalized weakness. The irregular and rapid heartbeat can lead to inefficient pumping of blood, compromising oxygen and nutrient delivery to the body's tissues. This can result in feelings of fatigue, decreased stamina, and reduced physical performance.

Shortness of Breath:

Atrial fibrillation can cause shortness of breath, especially during physical exertion or activities that increase the heart's workload. The compromised pumping function of the heart and the associated fluid buildup in the lungs can lead to a sensation of breathlessness or difficulty breathing.

Dizziness and Lightheadedness:

Some individuals with atrial fibrillation may experience episodes of dizziness or lightheadedness. The irregular heartbeat can affect blood flow to the brain, leading to temporary reductions in cerebral blood flow. This can result in feelings of dizziness, lightheadedness, or even fainting in severe cases.

Chest Discomfort:

Chest discomfort or chest pain is less commonly associated with atrial fibrillation but may occur, particularly if there are underlying heart conditions such as coronary artery disease or angina. The chest discomfort may range from mild to severe, and it is important to rule out other potential causes of chest pain.

Anxiety and Restlessness:

The irregular heartbeat and associated symptoms of atrial fibrillation can cause feelings of anxiety and restlessness in affected individuals. The awareness of a fast and irregular heart rhythm can be distressing and may lead to increased anxiety levels.

Reduced Exercise Tolerance:

Atrial fibrillation can significantly impact an individual's exercise tolerance. The irregular heartbeat, reduced cardiac output, and associated symptoms like fatigue and shortness of breath can limit physical activity and exercise capacity.

It is important to note that some individuals with atrial fibrillation may not experience any noticeable symptoms, a condition referred to as silent AF. However, even in the absence of symptoms, AF can still pose significant health risks, such as an increased risk of stroke. Regular medical check-ups and screenings are essential for identifying atrial fibrillation, particularly in high-risk individuals.

If any of these signs or symptoms are present, it is recommended to seek medical evaluation and consultation for proper diagnosis and appropriate management of atrial fibrillation. Early detection and intervention can help prevent complications and improve the quality of life for individuals with AF.

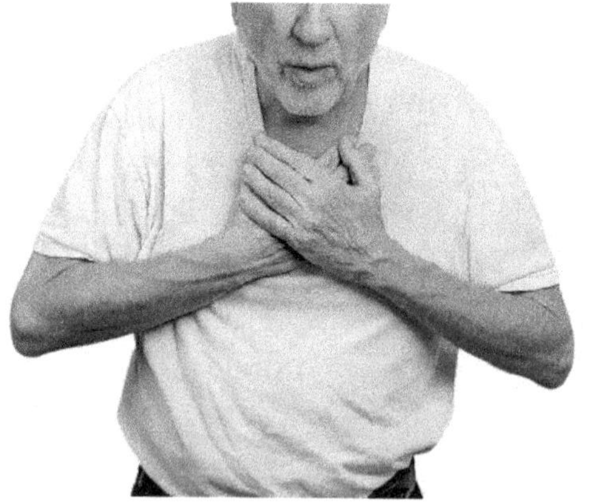

Importance of Timely Diagnosis and Monitoring

Timely diagnosis and ongoing monitoring of atrial fibrillation (AF) are crucial for several reasons. Prompt identification of AF allows for appropriate management strategies to be implemented, reducing the risk of complications and improving patient outcomes. Here are some key reasons highlighting the importance of timely diagnosis and monitoring of AF:

Risk of Stroke:

The risk of stroke is considerably increased by atrial fibrillation. The irregular and rapid heart rhythm in AF can lead to blood pooling in the atria, forming clots. A stroke may be brought on by a clot that breaks free and travels to the brain. Timely diagnosis enables the initiation of anticoagulant therapy, such as oral anticoagulants or blood thinners, to prevent clot formation and reduce the risk of stroke.

Symptom Management:

Timely diagnosis allows for the effective management of AF-related symptoms. Medications, lifestyle modifications, and other interventions can be initiated to control heart rate, restore normal heart rhythm, and alleviate symptoms such as palpitations, fatigue, shortness of breath, and dizziness. This leads to improved quality of life and overall well-being for individuals with AF.

Tailored Treatment Approach:

Each individual with AF may have different underlying causes, risk factors, and associated medical conditions. Timely diagnosis and ongoing monitoring enable healthcare professionals to tailor treatment plans specific to each patient's needs. This includes selecting appropriate medications, interventions, and lifestyle modifications based on the patient's unique circumstances, optimizing treatment outcomes and reducing the risk of complications.

Identification of Underlying Conditions:

Atrial fibrillation can be a manifestation of underlying medical conditions, such as hypertension, coronary artery disease, heart failure, or thyroid disorders. Timely diagnosis and monitoring of AF allow for the identification and evaluation of these underlying conditions. Treating and managing these underlying conditions not only helps in controlling AF but also improves overall cardiovascular health.

Evaluation of Treatment Efficacy:

Ongoing monitoring of AF enables healthcare professionals to evaluate the effectiveness of treatment interventions. Regular follow-up appointments, ECGs, and other monitoring methods help assess the patient's response to medications, identify any recurrences or complications, and make necessary adjustments to the treatment plan. This iterative approach ensures optimal management and helps in achieving long-term control of AF.

Prevention of Complications:

Timely diagnosis and monitoring of AF can help prevent or minimize the risk of complications associated with the condition. These complications may include the development of blood clots, heart failure, myocardial infarction, and other cardiovascular events. By closely monitoring the patient's heart rhythm, rate, and overall cardiovascular health, healthcare professionals can detect any abnormalities or signs of deterioration early on and take appropriate actions to prevent complications.

Patient Education and Empowerment:

Timely diagnosis provides an opportunity for healthcare providers to educate patients about their condition, including the causes, treatment options, and lifestyle modifications. By understanding their condition and actively participating in its management, patients can make informed decisions, implement necessary lifestyle changes, adhere to medications, and engage in self-monitoring practices. This empowers patients to take control of their health and contribute to the success of their treatment plan.

In conclusion, timely diagnosis and ongoing monitoring of atrial fibrillation are essential for optimizing patient outcomes, reducing the risk of complications, and improving the quality of life. Early detection allows for the implementation of appropriate treatment strategies, tailored to individual patients, while continuous monitoring ensures effective management, minimizes complications, and enhances long-term health outcomes for individuals with AF.

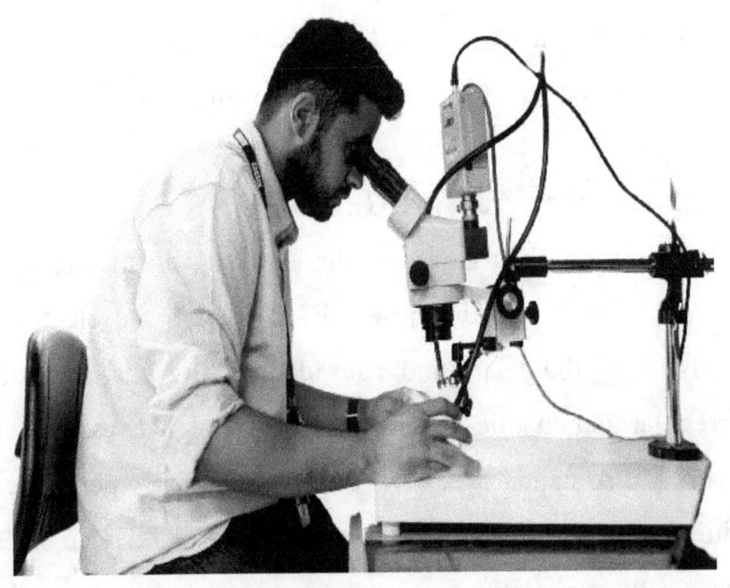

CHAPTER FOUR

Diagnostic Tools and Tests for Atrial Fibrillation

Accurate diagnosis of atrial fibrillation (AF) is essential for appropriate management and the prevention of complications. Healthcare providers employ a range of diagnostic tools and tests to confirm the presence of AF, determine its underlying causes, assess its severity, and guide treatment decisions. Let's explore some of the key diagnostic tools and tests used in the evaluation of AF:

1. Electrocardiogram (ECG):

The electrocardiogram is a fundamental diagnostic tool used to detect and diagnose AF. It records the electrical activity of the heart and can identify the characteristic irregular and chaotic pattern of electrical signals associated with AF. A standard 12-lead ECG is commonly performed during rest, but in some cases, a portable ECG device, such as a Holter monitor or event recorder, may be used for continuous or intermittent monitoring of the heart's electrical activity over an extended period.

2. Echocardiography:

Sound waves are used in echocardiography to provide live images of the heart. It offers helpful details regarding the makeup, operation, and blood flow of the heart. flow. The most popular kind, transthoracic echocardiography (TTE), is carried out by putting an ultrasound probe on the patient's chest. It can assess the size and function of the heart chambers, identify any structural abnormalities, evaluate the integrity of the heart valves, and estimate the ejection fraction (a measure of the heart's pumping efficiency). Transesophageal echocardiogram (TEE) involves the insertion of a flexible probe into the esophagus to obtain detailed images of the heart, particularly the atria and the presence of blood clots.

3. Cardiac Stress Tests:

Cardiac stress tests evaluate the heart's response to physical activity or medication-induced stress. These tests can help determine the presence of underlying coronary artery disease (CAD) or assess the heart's functional capacity.

Exercise stress tests involve using a treadmill or stationary bike while having your ECG monitored. Nuclear stress tests or stress echocardiography combine imaging techniques with stress testing to evaluate blood flow to the heart muscle during exercise or pharmacological stress.

4. Blood Tests:

Blood tests are commonly performed to assess various markers and conditions associated with AF. These may include blood tests to measure thyroid hormone levels (since thyroid dysfunction can contribute to AF), electrolyte levels (such as potassium, magnesium, and calcium), and specific biomarkers indicative of cardiac injury or stress (e.g., troponin). Additionally, blood tests can assess kidney and liver function, as these organs play a role in metabolizing medications used to manage AF.

5. Cardiac Imaging:

Advanced imaging techniques, such as cardiac computed tomography (CT) and cardiac magnetic resonance imaging (MRI), may be utilized to provide detailed images of the heart's structure and detect any underlying abnormalities.

These imaging modalities can help identify the presence of structural heart disease, evaluate the heart's chambers and valves, and assess for potential causes of AF, such as atrial enlargement or scar tissue.

6. Genetic Testing:

In some cases, genetic testing may be recommended to evaluate for specific genetic mutations or inherited conditions that can contribute to AF. This type of testing can help identify individuals at risk of developing AF at a younger age or with a family history of the condition.

It is important to note that the specific diagnostic tests and tools used may vary depending on the individual patient's symptoms, medical history, and clinical presentation. A comprehensive evaluation, including a detailed medical history, physical examination, and appropriate diagnostic tests, is essential to ensure an accurate diagnosis of AF and to guide the development of an individualized treatment plan.

By employing these diagnostic tools and tests, healthcare providers can accurately diagnose atrial fibrillation, assess its underlying causes and associated conditions, and tailor an appropriate management strategy. Early and accurate diagnosis enables prompt initiation of treatment, reducing the risk of complications and improving long-term outcomes for individuals with atrial fibrillation.

Electrocardiogram (ECG) and Other Imaging Techniques

Electrocardiogram (ECG) and other imaging techniques play a crucial role in the diagnosis and management of atrial fibrillation (AF). These tests provide valuable information about the heart's electrical activity, structure, and function, aiding in the accurate diagnosis, classification, and ongoing monitoring of AF. Here are the key imaging techniques commonly used in the evaluation of AF:

Electrocardiogram (ECG):

The electrical activity of the heart is measured using an electrocardiogram, a non-invasive diagnostic. It records the heart's rhythm and helps identify abnormal heartbeats, including atrial fibrillation. The characteristic findings on an ECG during AF include the absence of P waves, irregular R-R intervals, and fibrillatory waves (f waves) representing chaotic atrial electrical activity. ECG is an essential tool for diagnosing AF and assessing the heart's response to treatment interventions.

Holter Monitoring:

Holter monitoring is a type of ambulatory ECG monitoring that involves wearing a portable device that continuously records the heart's electrical activity for 24 to 48 hours or longer. It allows for prolonged monitoring of the heart rhythm, enabling the detection of intermittent or paroxysmal atrial fibrillation episodes that may not be captured during a standard ECG. Holter monitoring provides valuable information about the frequency, duration, and triggers of AF episodes, helping guide treatment decisions.

Event Monitoring:

Event monitoring is another type of ambulatory ECG monitoring that is used for longer-term monitoring of the heart's electrical activity. It is typically used when symptoms are infrequent or episodic. The device is activated by the patient when they experience symptoms, allowing for the recording of ECG during symptomatic episodes.

Event monitoring helps capture specific events related to AF, aiding in accurate diagnosis and guiding treatment decisions.

Echocardiography:

Echocardiography is an imaging technique that uses ultrasound waves to visualize the heart's structure and function. It provides valuable information about the size, shape, and function of the heart chambers, including the atria. Echocardiography can help identify structural abnormalities, such as valve disorders, left atrial enlargement, and other cardiac conditions that may contribute to atrial fibrillation. It also assesses the function of the heart and helps guide treatment strategies.

Cardiac Magnetic Resonance Imaging (MRI):

Cardiac MRI is a specialized imaging technique that provides detailed images of the heart's structure and function.

It can accurately assess the size and function of the heart chambers, identify any structural abnormalities, and evaluate blood flow patterns. Cardiac MRI is particularly useful in evaluating the underlying causes of atrial fibrillation, such as cardiomyopathies or congenital heart diseases. It helps guide treatment decisions and provides valuable information for risk stratification.

Computed Tomography (CT) Scan:

Computed tomography scanning uses X-rays and computer technology to create cross-sectional images of the heart. It is commonly used to assess the coronary arteries for the presence of any blockages or plaques that may contribute to atrial fibrillation. CT scans can also provide information about the heart's structure and help identify other potential causes or complications associated with AF. These imaging techniques, including ECG, holter monitoring, event monitoring, echocardiography, cardiac MRI, and CT scans, are invaluable tools in the diagnosis, classification, and ongoing monitoring of altrial fibrillation.

They provide important information about the heart's electrical activity, structure, and function, aiding in accurate diagnosis, risk stratification, and the development of personalized treatment plans. These imaging modalities are frequently used in combination to provide a comprehensive assessment of AF and guide clinical decision-making.

Holter Monitoring and Event Recorders

Holter monitoring and event recorders are specialized devices used for ambulatory electrocardiogram (ECG) monitoring. They play a crucial role in the diagnosis and management of atrial fibrillation (AF) by providing extended monitoring of the heart's electrical activity outside of a medical facility. These monitoring methods allow for the detection of intermittent or paroxysmal AF episodes that may not be captured during a standard ECG. Let's explore these techniques in detail:

Holter Monitoring:

Holter monitoring involves the use of a portable ECG device that is worn by the patient for an extended period, typically 24 to 48 hours or longer. The device continuously records the heart's electrical activity, capturing any abnormal rhythms or episodes of AF that may occur during daily activities. The collected data is then analyzed by healthcare professionals to identify and quantify AF episodes. Holter monitoring is particularly useful when symptoms are frequent or suspected AF episodes occur regularly.

Key features and benefits of Holter monitoring include:

a) Prolonged Monitoring: Holter monitoring allows for prolonged monitoring of the heart's electrical activity, providing a more comprehensive assessment compared to a standard ECG recording.

b) Symptom Correlation: Holter monitoring helps correlate symptoms experienced by the patient with recorded ECG abnormalities, aiding in the accurate diagnosis and characterization of AF episodes.

c) Detection of Silent AF: Silent AF refers to AF episodes that occur without noticeable symptoms. Holter monitoring can detect such episodes, allowing for timely intervention to prevent complications, such as stroke.

d) Assessment of Heart Rate Variability: Holter monitoring provides information about heart rate variability, which can be valuable in assessing autonomic nervous system function and identifying triggers for AF episodes.

e) Evaluation of Treatment Efficacy: Holter monitoring can assess the effectiveness of antiarrhythmic medications or other treatment interventions by monitoring changes in the frequency and duration of AF episodes over time.

Event Recorders:

Event recorders are small, portable devices that allow patients to record their ECG during symptomatic episodes or when they experience specific symptoms. These devices are typically used when symptoms are infrequent or episodic, making it challenging to capture them during routine clinic visits or continuous monitoring. Typically there are two types of event recorders:

a) Symptom-Activated Event Recorders: These recorders require the patient to manually activate the device when they experience symptoms. Once activated, the device records the ECG, capturing the heart's electrical activity during the symptomatic episode.

b) Automatic Event Recorders: Automatic event recorders continuously monitor the heart's electrical activity and automatically detect and record abnormal rhythms. These devices are particularly useful for detecting asymptomatic or unnoticed AF episodes.

Key features and benefits of event recorders include:

a) On-Demand Recording: Event recorders allow patients to record their ECG during episodes of symptoms, providing valuable data for accurate diagnosis and appropriate management.

b) Extended Monitoring: Event recorders provide the flexibility of extended monitoring, allowing patients to record their heart's electrical activity over a longer period if necessary.

c) Portability and Convenience: Event recorders are compact and portable, allowing patients to carry them with ease and record their ECG whenever necessary, even in their daily activities.

d) Data Transmission: Some event recorders have wireless or cellular connectivity, enabling the transmission of recorded data to healthcare providers for prompt analysis and interpretation.

e) Remote Monitoring: In certain cases, event recorders can be connected to remote monitoring systems, where healthcare professionals can access the recorded data in real-time, providing timely feedback and intervention if required.

Holter monitoring and event recorders are valuable tools in the diagnosis and management of atrial fibrillation. They provide extended monitoring of the heart's electrical activity, allowing for the detection of intermittent or paroxysmal AF episodes, correlation of symptoms, evaluation of treatment efficacy, and assessment of heart rate variability.

These monitoring techniques enhance diagnostic accuracy, guide treatment decisions, and ultimately improve patient outcomes in the management of AF.

Blood Tests and Biomarkers

Blood tests and biomarkers are essential tools in the evaluation and management of atrial fibrillation (AF). They provide valuable information about various physiological and biochemical markers that can aid in diagnosing AF, assessing its underlying causes, determining treatment strategies, and monitoring the condition. Let's delve into the details of blood tests and biomarkers commonly used in AF:

Complete Blood Count (CBC):

A complete blood count measures the levels of different blood cells, including red blood cells, white blood cells, and platelets. While a CBC may not directly diagnose AF, it can help identify underlying conditions that may contribute to AF, such as anemia or infection.

Anemia can lead to a higher risk of AF, and treating it can improve AF management.

Thyroid Function Tests:

Thyroid function tests measure the levels of thyroid hormones in the blood, including thyroid-stimulating hormone (TSH), free thyroxine (FT4), and triiodothyronine (T3). Thyroid disorders, such as hyperthyroidism or hypothyroidism, can contribute to the development or exacerbation of AF. Evaluating thyroid function helps identify and manage these underlying conditions.

Cardiac Biomarkers:

Cardiac biomarkers are substances released into the bloodstream in response to cardiac injury or stress. While not specific to AF, they can provide information about associated cardiac conditions or complications. Common cardiac biomarkers include troponin, creatine kinase-MB (CK-MB), and brain natriuretic peptide (BNP).

Elevated levels of these biomarkers may indicate cardiac damage, such as myocardial infarction or heart failure, which can occur in conjunction with AF.

Coagulation Profile:

Coagulation profile tests, such as prothrombin time (PT) and international normalized ratio (INR), assess the blood's clotting ability. Since AF increases the risk of blood clot formation, evaluating the coagulation profile helps determine the need for anticoagulant therapy to prevent stroke and other thromboembolic complications.

Renal Function Tests:

Renal function tests, including blood urea nitrogen (BUN) and creatinine levels assess the kidney's ability to filter waste products from the blood. Impaired renal function may impact medication clearance and dosage adjustments, which is important when prescribing anticoagulants or antiarrhythmic drugs for AF management.

Inflammatory Markers:

Inflammatory markers, such as C-reactive protein (CRP) and erythrocyte sedimentation rate (ESR), help evaluate the presence and extent of systemic inflammation. Inflammation can contribute to the development and progression of AF. Monitoring inflammatory markers can aid in risk assessment, identifying potential triggers, and guiding treatment strategies.

Genetic Testing:

Genetic testing is not routinely performed for AF but may be considered in specific cases, particularly when a genetic predisposition is suspected. Certain genetic mutations can increase the risk of developing AF or alter the response to certain medications. Genetic testing can provide valuable insights into the underlying mechanisms of AF and assist in personalized treatment approaches.

Electrolyte Levels:

Measurement of electrolyte levels, including potassium (K+), magnesium (Mg2+), and calcium (Ca2+), is essential in AF management. Imbalances in electrolytes can disrupt the heart's electrical conduction system and trigger or perpetuate AF. Monitoring and correcting electrolyte imbalances are crucial in maintaining a stable cardiac rhythm and optimizing the efficacy of antiarrhythmic therapies.

The use of blood tests and biomarkers in AF helps healthcare professionals assess the overall health status, identify underlying conditions, and evaluate the risk of complications, guide treatment decisions, and monitor treatment efficacy.

These tests complement other diagnostic methods and provide valuable information for a comprehensive understanding of an individual's AF condition. Integrating blood tests and biomarkers into the management of AF enables personalized care and improves patient outcomes.

Echocardiography and Transesophageal Echocardiogram (TEE)

Echocardiography and transesophageal echocardiogram (TEE) are important imaging techniques used in the evaluation and management of atrial fibrillation (AF). These tests provide detailed information about the structure and function of the heart, allowing healthcare professionals to assess the underlying causes of AF, determine treatment strategies, and monitor the condition. Let's explore these imaging modalities in detail:

Echocardiography:

Use of ultrasonic waves to provide in-the-moment images of the heart is known as echocardiography. It provides valuable information about the size, shape, and function of the heart chambers, including the atria. Echocardiography allows for the assessment of various parameters relevant to AF, such as left atrial size and function, presence of structural abnormalities, and the overall function of the heart.

Key features and benefits of echocardiography include:

a) Assessment of Atrial Function: Echocardiography enables the evaluation of atrial function, including atrial contraction and relaxation, which is essential in understanding the mechanisms and consequences of AF.

b) Detection of Structural Abnormalities: Echocardiography helps identify structural abnormalities that may contribute to AF, such as mitral valve disease, left atrial enlargement, or congenital heart defects. Identifying these abnormalities aids in the selection of appropriate treatment strategies.

c) Determination of Ejection Fraction: Echocardiography provides information about the heart's ejection fraction, which is a measure of the heart's pumping function. Changes in ejection fraction can occur in individuals with AF and may impact treatment decisions and prognosis.

d) Guidance for Cardioversion: Echocardiography helps assess the presence of blood clots in the atria before considering electrical cardioversion. This evaluation is crucial to avoid the risk of embolic events, such as strokes.

e) Monitoring Treatment Response: Echocardiography is valuable in monitoring the response to treatment interventions, such as medications or procedures. It can assess changes in atrial size, function, and overall cardiac performance over time.

Transesophageal Echocardiogram (TEE):

Transesophageal echocardiogram (TEE) is a specialized type of echocardiography that provides more detailed images of the heart's structures, particularly the atria, by inserting a small ultrasound probe into the esophagus. TEE is particularly useful in assessing the presence of blood clots in the left atrium or left atrial appendage, which can pose a significant risk of embolization during certain procedures or in patients with AF.

Key features and benefits of TEE include:

a) Detection of Atrial Thrombus: TEE offers better visualization of the left atrial appendage and can accurately assess the presence or absence of blood clots. This information is crucial in determining the safety of procedures, such as cardioversion or atrial appendage occlusion, and guiding the use of anticoagulant therapy.

b) High-Resolution Imaging: TEE provides higher resolution images compared to transthoracic echocardiography, allowing for more precise assessment of atrial structures, valve function, and potential sources of emboli.

c) Evaluation of Atrial Septum: TEE allows for detailed evaluation of the atrial septum, which is important in detecting potential defects or abnormalities that may contribute to AF.

d) Guidance for Catheter Ablation: TEE can assist during catheter ablation procedures by providing real-time visualization of the catheter's position and the surrounding structures, ensuring safe and effective ablation of the targeted areas.

e) Preoperative Assessment: TEE is often used in preoperative evaluations for cardiac surgery, providing detailed information about the heart's structures and function, allowing surgeons to plan and optimize the surgical approach.

Echocardiography and TEE are indispensable imaging tools in the management of AF. They provide valuable information about atrial structure, function, and the presence of blood clots, assisting in diagnosis, treatment selection, and procedural guidance. These non-invasive techniques aid in the personalized management of AF, improve patient outcomes, and contribute to a comprehensive understanding of the underlying cardiovascular conditions associated with AF.

CHAPTER FIVE

Complications and Consequences of Atrial Fibrillation

Atrial fibrillation (AF) is not just an irregular heart rhythm; it can have significant implications for a person's health and well-being. If left untreated or poorly managed, AF can lead to various complications and consequences. Understanding these potential outcomes is crucial in highlighting the importance of proper management and timely interventions. Let's explore some of the common complications and consequences associated with AF:

1. Stroke: One of the most serious complications of AF is the increased risk of stroke. AF disrupts the normal blood flow in the atria, leading to the formation of blood clots. These clots can travel to the brain and block blood vessels, causing an ischemic stroke.

In fact, individuals with AF have a fivefold higher risk of stroke compared to those without AF. Stroke prevention strategies, such as anticoagulant medications, are often prescribed to reduce the risk of blood clot formation.

2. Heart Failure: AF can contribute to the development or exacerbation of heart failure, a condition in which the heart is unable to pump blood effectively. The irregular and rapid heart rhythm in AF compromises the heart's ability to fill and empty properly, leading to inadequate blood supply to the body's organs and tissues. Treating and managing AF is crucial in preventing or minimizing the progression of heart failure.

3. Impaired Quality of Life: The symptoms associated with AF, such as palpitations, fatigue, shortness of breath, and reduced exercise tolerance, can significantly impact a person's quality of life. AF-related symptoms may limit daily activities, affect sleep patterns, and lead to emotional distress.

Effective management of AF, including symptom control and rhythm management can improve quality of life and restore functional capacity.

4. Increased Mortality: AF is associated with an increased risk of mortality, particularly due to its association with stroke, heart failure, and other cardiovascular complications. Timely and appropriate management of AF, including stroke prevention strategies and controlling underlying risk factors, can help reduce the risk of premature death.

5. Cardiovascular Events: AF is linked to an increased risk of other cardiovascular events, such as myocardial infarction (heart attack) and peripheral arterial disease. The irregular heart rhythm and compromised blood flow associated with AF can contribute to the development or worsening of these conditions. Effective management of AF, alongside optimal control of other cardiovascular risk factors, can help reduce the incidence of such events.

6. Cognitive Impairment: There is emerging evidence suggesting a link between AF and cognitive impairment, including an increased risk of dementia and decline in cognitive function. The mechanisms underlying this association are not yet fully understood, but factors such as reduced cerebral blood flow, microemboli from the heart, and inflammation may contribute. Timely detection and management of AF, along with addressing modifiable risk factors, may help reduce the risk of cognitive decline.

7. Worsening of Underlying Conditions: AF can worsen the symptoms and outcomes of other underlying medical conditions, such as hypertension, coronary artery disease, and valvular heart disease. The irregular heart rhythm and hemodynamic changes associated with AF can place additional strain on the heart and exacerbate the progression of these conditions. Treating and controlling AF is crucial in preventing the worsening of underlying cardiovascular diseases.

It is important to emphasize that the risk and severity of complications and consequences can vary among individuals with AF. Factors such as the presence of underlying medical conditions, the duration and frequency of AF episodes, and the effectiveness of treatment strategies can influence outcomes. Regular medical follow-ups, adherence to prescribed medications, and lifestyle modifications are essential in minimizing the risk of complications and optimizing overall cardiovascular health.

By addressing these potential complications and consequences of AF, healthcare providers can emphasize the importance of early diagnosis, comprehensive management, and regular monitoring to improve patient outcomes and boost their overall quality of life.

Increased Stroke and Thromboembolism Risk in Atrial Fibrillation

Atrial fibrillation (AF) poses a significant risk for stroke and thromboembolism, making stroke prevention a vital aspect of managing this cardiac arrhythmia. AF disrupts the normal blood flow in the atria, leading to the formation of blood clots that can travel to the brain and cause an ischemic stroke. Understanding the increased risk of stroke and thromboembolism in AF is crucial in implementing appropriate preventive strategies. Let's explore this crucial feature in more detail:

1. Thrombus Formation: In AF, the irregular and rapid electrical signals in the atria can cause blood to pool or stagnate, particularly in the left atrial appendage (LAA), a small pouch in the heart. This stagnant blood may form clots, or thrombi, within the LAA. These thrombi have the potential to dislodge and travel through the bloodstream, leading to embolism.

2. Embolic Stroke: When a blood clot (embolus) travels from the heart to the brain and obstructs a blood vessel, it results in an embolic stroke. The clot can block the blood flow to a specific region of the brain, leading to ischemia and subsequent neurological deficits. Embolic strokes associated with AF tend to be more severe and have a higher mortality rate compared to strokes from other causes.

3. CHA2DS2-VASc Score: To assess the risk of stroke in individuals with AF, healthcare providers often use a risk stratification tool called the CHA2DS2-VASc score. This scoring system evaluates various clinical factors, including age, sex, presence of heart failure, hypertension, diabetes, prior stroke or transient ischemic attack (TIA), vascular disease, and the presence of other comorbidities. The score helps determine the need for anticoagulant therapy for stroke prevention.

4. Anticoagulation Therapy: Anticoagulation therapy plays a pivotal role in reducing the risk of stroke and thromboembolism in AF patients. The use of anticoagulants aims to prevent the formation of blood clots and inhibit clotting factors. Vitamin K antagonists (e.g., warfarin) and direct oral anticoagulants (DOACs) such as dabigatran, rivaroxaban, apixaban, and edoxaban are commonly prescribed medications. The choice of anticoagulant depends on factors such as patient characteristics, bleeding risk, and drug interactions.

5. Left Atrial Appendage Closure: In some cases, individuals with AF who are at high risk of stroke and have contraindications to long-term anticoagulation therapy may be considered for left atrial appendage closure (LAAC). This minimally invasive procedure involves sealing off the LAA to prevent blood clot formation. LAAC can be performed surgically or through catheter-based approaches, such as the use of a device called the Watchman.

6. Risk Factor Modification: Managing underlying risk factors associated with stroke can further reduce the risk in AF patients. Blood pressure control, glycemic control in diabetes, lipid management, and lifestyle modifications such as regular exercise, maintaining a healthy weight, and avoiding smoking are important strategies to mitigate the risk of stroke.

7. Shared Decision-Making: The decision regarding stroke prevention strategies in AF should be made through shared decision-making between the patient and healthcare provider. Factors such as the individual's overall health status, bleeding risk, compliance with medications, and patient preferences should be taken into account to determine the most appropriate stroke prevention approach.

It is important to note that not all individuals with AF have the same risk of stroke, and the decision for anticoagulation therapy should be based on an individualized assessment.

Regular monitoring, adherence to medication regimens and periodic re-evaluation of stroke risk are essential to ensure optimal stroke prevention strategies.

By understanding the increased risk of stroke and thromboembolism in atrial fibrillation and implementing appropriate preventive measures, healthcare providers can significantly reduce the occurrence of devastating strokes and improve the long-term outcomes for individuals with AF.

Heart Failure and Cardiac Remodeling in Atrial Fibrillation

Atrial fibrillation (AF) and heart failure often coexist and can significantly impact each other's progression and outcomes. The irregular and rapid electrical signals in AF can lead to changes in the structure and function of the heart, a process known as cardiac remodeling.

Understanding the relationship between AF, heart failure, and cardiac remodeling is crucial in managing these conditions effectively. Let's explore the details of heart failure and cardiac remodeling in the context of AF:

1. Heart Failure and AF: Heart failure occurs when the heart is unable to pump blood efficiently, leading to inadequate circulation of oxygen and nutrients to the body's organs and tissues. AF can contribute to the development or worsening of heart failure by several mechanisms. The irregular and rapid heart rhythm in AF compromises the heart's ability to fill and contract effectively, reducing its overall pumping capacity. This can lead to symptoms such as fatigue, shortness of breath, fluid retention, and exercise intolerance.

2. Systolic and Diastolic Dysfunction: AF can cause both systolic and diastolic dysfunction, affecting the heart's ability to contract and relax properly.

Systolic dysfunction refers to the impaired ability of the heart to pump blood out effectively during each contraction, while diastolic dysfunction refers to impaired relaxation and filling of the heart during the resting phase. Both types of dysfunction can contribute to the development of heart failure.

3. Structural Changes: Prolonged and uncontrolled AF can lead to structural changes in the heart, such as atrial dilation, ventricular remodeling, and fibrosis. Atrial dilation occurs when the atria enlarge due to the irregular and rapid electrical activity, which can lead to further electrical instability and perpetuation of AF. Ventricular remodeling involves changes in the size, shape, and function of the ventricles, potentially impairing their pumping ability. Fibrosis, the accumulation of scar tissue, can occur in both the atria and ventricles, further disrupting the normal electrical and mechanical function of the heart.

4. Neurohormonal Activation: AF and heart failure trigger a cascade of neurohormonal responses, including the activation of the renin-angiotensin-aldosterone system (RAAS) and sympathetic nervous system. These responses aim to compensate for the reduced cardiac output but can contribute to further cardiac remodeling. Chronic activation of the RAAS and sympathetic pathways can promote inflammation, fibrosis, and vasoconstriction, exacerbating the structural and functional changes in the heart.

5. Impact on Treatment and Prognosis: The presence of heart failure in individuals with AF can influence treatment strategies and prognosis. Effective management of heart failure, including optimizing medication regimens, controlling fluid balance, and addressing underlying causes, is essential in improving symptoms and outcomes. In some cases, interventions such as cardiac resynchronization therapy (CRT) or implantable cardioverter-defibrillator (ICD) placement may be considered.

Additionally, the coexistence of heart failure can affect the choice and dosing of antiarrhythmic medications or anticoagulant therapy for AF.

6. Shared Risk Factors: AF and heart failure often share common risk factors such as hypertension, coronary artery disease, valvular heart disease, obesity, and diabetes. Addressing these modifiable risk factors through lifestyle modifications, medication therapy, and appropriate interventions is crucial in managing both AF and heart failure and mitigating their detrimental effects on the heart.

7. Multidisciplinary Approach: Given the complex interplay between AF, heart failure, and cardiac remodeling, a multidisciplinary approach involving cardiologists, electrophysiologists, heart failure specialists, and other healthcare professionals is essential.

Collaboration among these experts helps optimize treatment strategies, monitor disease progression, and provide comprehensive care to individuals with AF and heart failure.

By recognizing the relationship between AF, heart failure, and cardiac remodeling, healthcare providers can tailor management strategies to address the specific needs of each patient. Early detection, aggressive risk factor management, appropriate medication therapy, and regular monitoring are key elements in improving outcomes and quality of life for individuals with AF and heart failure.

Impact on Quality of Life and Daily Functioning in Atrial Fibrillation

Atrial fibrillation (AF) is a chronic condition that can significantly impact an individual's quality of life and daily functioning. The symptoms, treatment requirements, and psychological effects of living with AF can affect various aspects of a person's well-being.

Understanding the impact of AF on quality of life is crucial in providing comprehensive care to individuals with this cardiac arrhythmia. Let's explore the details of how AF can affect quality of life and daily functioning:

1. Symptoms: AF can cause a range of symptoms that can significantly impair daily functioning and quality of life. Common symptoms include palpitations, shortness of breath, fatigue, dizziness, chest discomfort, and reduced exercise tolerance. These symptoms can limit physical activities, impact social interactions, and lead to emotional distress.

2. Activity Limitations: The symptoms and unpredictability of AF can result in limitations in physical activities and exercise. Individuals may feel apprehensive about engaging in activities that may trigger or worsen AF episodes. This can lead to a sedentary lifestyle, decreased fitness levels, and reduced overall well-being.

3. Emotional Impact: Living with a chronic condition like AF can have a significant emotional toll. Individuals may experience anxiety, fear, frustration, and a sense of loss of control over their health. The uncertainty surrounding AF, the need for ongoing medical management, and the potential for complications can contribute to psychological distress and affect mental well-being.

4. Sleep Disturbances: AF can disrupt sleep patterns, leading to poor sleep quality and daytime fatigue. Sleep disturbances can further impact daily functioning, concentration, and overall productivity.

5. Treatment Burden: Managing AF often involves a complex treatment regimen, including medication adherence, lifestyle modifications, regular medical appointments, and possible interventions such as cardioversion or catheter ablation. The treatment burden can affect individuals' daily routines, financial resources, and overall well-being.

6. Social Impact: AF can also have social implications. The unpredictable nature of AF episodes may require individuals to make lifestyle adjustments and avoid certain activities or social events. This can lead to feelings of isolation, reduced participation in social activities, and challenges in maintaining relationships.

7. Cognitive Function: Studies suggest that AF may be associated with cognitive impairment and an increased risk of stroke-related cognitive decline. Cognitive difficulties can impact memory, concentration, and overall cognitive function, affecting daily activities and quality of life.

8. Psychological Support: The psychological impact of AF should not be underestimated. Providing adequate psychological support, education, and resources can help individuals cope with the emotional challenges associated with living with AF. Support groups, counseling, and stress management techniques can be beneficial in improving overall well-being.

9. Shared Decision-Making: Involving individuals with AF in shared decision-making regarding their treatment options, lifestyle modifications, and self-care empowers them to actively participate in their healthcare. This collaborative approach helps tailor the management plan to the individual's preferences, values, and goals, ultimately improving their quality of life.

10. Holistic Care: Taking a holistic approach to AF management is essential. This entails addressing well-being in terms of the physical, emotional, and social spheres. Integrating physical activity, stress reduction techniques, adequate sleep, and promoting healthy lifestyle choices can have a positive impact on quality of life and daily functioning.

By recognizing and addressing the impact of AF on quality of life and daily functioning, healthcare providers can provide comprehensive care that not only focuses on managing the physical aspects of AF but also improves overall well-being and enhances the individual's ability to lead a fulfilling life.

CHAPTER SIX

Preventive Measures in Atrial Fibrillation

Preventing the onset or progression of atrial fibrillation (AF) is a crucial aspect of managing this cardiac arrhythmia. By implementing preventive measures, individuals can reduce their risk of developing AF or experiencing recurrent episodes. Additionally, preventive strategies play a vital role in minimizing complications associated with AF and improving overall cardiovascular health. Let's explore the details of preventive measures in atrial fibrillation:

1. Lifestyle Modifications:

a. Maintain a Healthy Weight: Excess weight and obesity can increase the risk of developing AF. By achieving and maintaining a healthy weight through a balanced diet and regular physical activity, individuals can reduce their risk of AF.

b. Adopt a Heart-Healthy Diet: A diet rich in fruits, vegetables, whole grains, lean proteins, and low-fat dairy products is beneficial for cardiovascular health.

Limiting the intake of saturated fats, cholesterol, sodium, and refined sugars can help prevent AF.

c. Engage in Regular Physical Activity: Regular exercise contributes to overall cardiovascular health and can help prevent AF. Aim to complete 75 minutes of vigorous aerobic exercise or 150 minutes of moderate aerobic exercise each week.

d. Manage Stress: Chronic stress can contribute to the development and progression of AF. Implement stress-reduction techniques such as meditation, deep breathing exercises, yoga, or engaging in hobbies to promote overall well-being and reduce the risk of AF.

e. Limit Alcohol Consumption: Excessive alcohol consumption is associated with an increased risk of AF.

It is advisable to limit alcohol intake to moderate levels or abstain from alcohol altogether, depending on individual circumstances.

f. Quit Smoking: Smoking is a significant risk factor for AF and other cardiovascular diseases. Quitting smoking significantly reduces the risk of developing AF and improves overall cardiovascular health.

2. Blood Pressure Management:

a. Maintain Optimal Blood Pressure: High blood pressure (hypertension) is a significant risk factor for AF. Regular monitoring of blood pressure and effective management through lifestyle modifications and medication therapy, if necessary, can help prevent AF.

3. Diabetes Management:

a. Control Blood Sugar Levels: Individuals with diabetes have an increased risk of developing AF.

Effective management of diabetes, including maintaining stable blood sugar levels through diet, exercise, and medication as prescribed, can help prevent AF.

4. Management of Other Underlying Medical Conditions:

a. Control Thyroid Disorders: Thyroid disorders, such as hyperthyroidism, can contribute to the development of AF. Adequate management of thyroid function through medication and regular monitoring can help prevent AF.

b. Manage Obstructive Sleep Apnea: Obstructive sleep apnea (OSA) is associated with an increased risk of AF. Treating OSA with continuous positive airway pressure (CPAP) therapy or other interventions can reduce the risk of AF.

c. Address Structural Heart Diseases: Structural heart diseases, such as valvular heart disease or congenital heart defects, can predispose individuals to AF. Effective management and treatment of these underlying conditions can help prevent AF.

5. Medication Therapy:

a. Anticoagulation Therapy: For individuals with AF at increased risk of stroke, anticoagulant medications may be prescribed to reduce the risk of blood clots and stroke.

b. Antiarrhythmic Medications: In certain cases, antiarrhythmic medications may be prescribed to maintain normal heart rhythm and prevent AF episodes.

6. Regular Medical Follow-up:

a. Regular Check-ups: Routine medical follow-up appointments allow healthcare providers to monitor the individual's condition, assess treatment effectiveness, and make necessary adjustments to preventive measures and medication therapy.

b. Health Education: Providing individuals with AF with adequate health education about their condition, preventive measures, medication adherence, and recognizing potential triggers can empower them to actively participate in their care and prevent AF-related complications.

By implementing these preventive measures, individuals can significantly reduce their risk of developing AF, minimize the frequency and severity of AF episodes, and improve overall cardiovascular health. However, it is essential to consult with a healthcare provider for personalized recommendations based on individual risk factors, medical history, and specific needs.

Lifestyle Modifications for Atrial Fibrillation Prevention

Making certain lifestyle modifications plays a crucial role in preventing the onset or progression of atrial fibrillation (AF). By adopting healthy habits and minimizing certain risk factors, individuals can significantly reduce their risk of developing AF or experiencing recurrent episodes. Lifestyle modifications are particularly important for individuals with known risk factors for AF or those who have already been diagnosed with this cardiac arrhythmia. Let's explore the details of lifestyle modifications for AF prevention:

1. Maintain a Healthy Weight:

Maintaining a healthy weight is essential for reducing the risk of developing AF. Excess weight and obesity increase the strain on the heart and can contribute to cardiovascular issues. By achieving and maintaining a healthy weight through a balanced diet and regular exercise, individuals can lower their risk of AF.

It is recommended to consult with a healthcare provider or registered dietitian for personalized guidance on appropriate calorie intake, portion sizes, and specific dietary recommendations.

2. Adopt a Heart-Healthy Diet:

A heart-healthy diet is crucial for cardiovascular health and AF prevention. Focus on consuming a variety of nutrient-rich foods, including fruits, vegetables, whole grains, lean proteins (such as fish and poultry), and low-fat dairy products. Minimize the intake of saturated fats, trans fats, cholesterol, sodium, and added sugars. Avoid using frying as a cooking method and choose grilling, baking, or steaming instead. Following a heart-healthy diet can help maintain proper blood pressure, cholesterol levels, and overall heart function.

3. Engage in Regular Physical Activity:

Regular exercise is beneficial for overall cardiovascular health and can help prevent AF.

Spend at least 150 minutes per week participating in moderate-intensity aerobic exercises such brisk walking, swimming, cycling, or dancing. Alternatively, vigorous-intensity activities like jogging, running, or aerobic classes can be performed for 75 minutes per week. Additionally, include muscle-strengthening activities on two or more days per week, focusing on major muscle groups. However, it is important to consult with a healthcare provider before starting any exercise program, especially if there are existing health conditions or concerns.

4. Manage Stress:

Chronic stress can contribute to the development and progression of AF. Implementing stress management techniques can be beneficial in AF prevention. Explore stress reduction methods such as mindfulness meditation, deep breathing exercises, yoga, tai chi, or engaging in hobbies that promote relaxation. Find activities that help relieve stress and create a sense of calm and well-being. Adequate sleep, regular exercise, and maintaining a healthy work-life balance are also crucial in managing stress levels.

5. Limit Alcohol Consumption:

Alcoholism in excess is a proven risk factor for AF. It is recommended to limit alcohol intake to moderate levels or abstain from alcohol altogether, depending on individual circumstances. Excessive alcohol intake can disrupt the heart's electrical signals and trigger AF episodes.

6. Quit Smoking:

Smoking is a significant risk factor for AF and other cardiovascular diseases. Quitting smoking is crucial for preventing AF and improving overall cardiovascular health. Seek support from healthcare providers, use smoking cessation aids, join smoking cessation programs, or seek counseling to quit smoking successfully. Even if you have smoked for many years, quitting can still provide significant benefits to your heart health.

7. Maintain Blood Pressure and Cholesterol Levels:

High blood pressure (hypertension) and high cholesterol levels can increase the risk of developing AF. It is important to regularly monitor blood pressure and cholesterol levels and manage them within recommended ranges. Lifestyle modifications, such as a heart-healthy diet, regular exercise, weight management, limiting sodium intake, and avoiding tobacco smoke, can help maintain optimal blood pressure and cholesterol levels.

8 Manage Diabetes:

Diabetes is a risk factor for AF, and effective management of blood sugar levels is crucial. It is important to follow a well-balanced diet, engage in regular physical activity, monitor blood sugar levels as recommended by healthcare providers, take prescribed medications as directed, and attend regular check-ups to effectively manage diabetes and prevent AF.

9. Seek Regular Medical Check-ups:

Regular medical check-ups are important for assessing overall health and identifying any potential risk factors or underlying conditions that may contribute to AF. Follow the recommended schedule for routine check-ups, blood pressure monitoring, and other necessary screenings. Regular follow-up with healthcare providers allows for early detection and management of any emerging health concerns.

By incorporating these lifestyle modifications, individuals can significantly reduce their risk of developing AF and improve overall cardiovascular health. However, it is important to consult with a healthcare provider for personalized recommendations based on individual risk factors, medical history, and specific needs. Taking proactive steps towards a heart-healthy lifestyle can lead to long-term benefits in AF prevention and overall well-being.

Managing Underlying Health Conditions in Atrial Fibrillation

Atrial fibrillation (AF) often coexists with underlying health conditions, and effectively managing these conditions is essential for optimal management of AF. By addressing and controlling underlying health conditions, individuals with AF can reduce the frequency and severity of AF episodes, lower the risk of complications, and improve overall cardiovascular health. Let's explore the details of managing common underlying health conditions associated with AF:

1. Hypertension (High Blood Pressure):
Controlling blood pressure is crucial in managing AF. Lifestyle modifications play a key role, including maintaining a healthy weight, following a heart-healthy diet, reducing sodium intake, exercising regularly, limiting alcohol consumption, managing stress, and quitting smoking. Additionally, medication therapy may be prescribed by healthcare providers to help manage blood pressure levels effectively.

2. Coronary Artery Disease (CAD):

CAD occurs when the blood vessels that supply the heart muscle with oxygen-rich blood become narrowed or blocked due to the buildup of plaque. Managing CAD involves lifestyle modifications, such as adopting a heart-healthy diet, engaging in regular physical activity, managing blood pressure and cholesterol levels, quitting smoking, and taking prescribed medications (such as antiplatelet agents, beta-blockers, and statins) to reduce the risk of further complications.

3. Heart Failure:

Heart failure ensues when the heart is unable to pump blood efficiently. Managing heart failure in the presence of AF requires a comprehensive approach. This may include lifestyle modifications such as following a low-sodium diet, managing fluid intake, regular physical activity as recommended by healthcare providers, and taking prescribed medications (such as diuretics, ACE inhibitors, beta-blockers, and/or angiotensin receptor blockers) to optimize heart function and control symptoms.

4. Diabetes:

Effective management of diabetes is essential in individuals with AF. This involves maintaining stable blood sugar levels through lifestyle modifications, including following a balanced diet, engaging in regular physical activity, monitoring blood sugar levels as recommended by healthcare providers, taking prescribed medications (such as oral hypoglycemic agents or insulin), and attending regular check-ups to monitor and adjust treatment as necessary.

5. Thyroid Disorders:

Managing underlying thyroid disorders, such as hyperthyroidism or hypothyroidism, is important in AF management. Treatment approaches may vary depending on the specific thyroid disorder and individual circumstances. Medication therapy, radioactive iodine therapy, or surgical interventions may be prescribed to achieve and maintain proper thyroid hormone levels.

6. Obstructive Sleep Apnea (OSA):

 OSA is a common comorbidity with AF and can contribute to its development and progression. Effective management of OSA may involve lifestyle modifications, such as weight loss, avoiding alcohol and sedatives, and using continuous positive airway pressure (CPAP) therapy. CPAP therapy helps keep the airway open during sleep and reduces the risk of breathing disturbances that can trigger AF episodes.

7. Valvular Heart Disease:

 Managing underlying valvular heart disease is essential for individuals with AF. Treatment approaches may vary depending on the specific valvular condition and its severity. Medication therapy, heart valve repair, or heart valve replacement surgery may be recommended to address the underlying valvular abnormality and optimize heart function.

8. Other Underlying Health Conditions:

Depending on individual circumstances, other underlying health conditions such as chronic kidney disease, lung diseases, anemia, and certain genetic disorders may require specific management strategies.

Collaboration with healthcare providers who specialize in the respective areas is important to ensure comprehensive care and management of these conditions in conjunction with AF.

It is important for individuals with AF to work closely with their healthcare providers to develop a personalized treatment plan that addresses their underlying health conditions. Regular follow-up appointments, adherence to prescribed medications and lifestyle modifications, and open communication with healthcare providers are crucial for effectively managing these conditions and reducing the burden of AF. With proper management of underlying health conditions, individuals with AF can enhance their overall well-being and improve their quality of life.

Medications and Anticoagulation Therapy in Atrial Fibrillation

Medications play a vital role in the management of atrial fibrillation (AF). The primary goals of medication therapy in AF are to control heart rate, restore and maintain normal heart rhythm (sinus rhythm), and reduce the risk of complications, particularly stroke and systemic embolism. Additionally, anticoagulation therapy is often prescribed to prevent blood clot formation. Let's delve into the details of commonly used medications and anticoagulation therapy in AF:

1. Rate Control Medications:

Rate control medications aim to regulate the heart rate in individuals with AF by slowing down the electrical signals that pass through the atria to the ventricles. Commonly prescribed rate control medications include beta-blockers (such as metoprolol, atenolol), calcium channel blockers (such as diltiazem, verapamil), and digitalis preparations (such as digoxin).

These medications help control the heart rate during AF, alleviate symptoms, and improve overall cardiovascular function.

2. Rhythm Control Medications:

Rhythm control medications are used to restore and maintain normal heart rhythm (sinus rhythm) in individuals with AF. They function by reducing the heart's aberrant electrical signals. Antiarrhythmic medications are often prescribed for rhythm control, including class I agents (such as flecainide, propafenone), class III agents (such as amiodarone, sotalol), and sometimes class IC agents (such as dofetilide). These medications are typically initiated under close medical supervision and their selection depends on various factors, including the presence of structural heart disease and individual patient characteristics.

3. Anticoagulation Therapy:

Anticoagulation therapy is a critical component of AF management to prevent blood clot formation and reduce the risk of stroke and systemic embolism.

The decision to prescribe anticoagulants is based on an individual's risk factors for stroke, as assessed by scoring systems such as CHA2DS2-VASc. The two primary categories of anticoagulants are:

a. Vitamin K Antagonists (VKAs): Medications such as warfarin are traditional oral anticoagulants that have been used for many years. VKAs require regular blood monitoring to maintain the appropriate level of anticoagulation, as measured by the international normalized ratio (INR).

b. Direct Oral Anticoagulants (DOACs): DOACs, including rivaroxaban, apixaban, dabigatran, and edoxaban, are newer oral anticoagulants that offer a more convenient dosing regimen and do not require routine blood monitoring. DOACs have shown comparable or superior efficacy and safety to VKAs and are the preferred choice for most individuals with AF.

The selection of anticoagulant therapy is based on individual patient characteristics, including age, renal function, bleeding risk, and concomitant medications. It is crucial to discuss the benefits and risks of anticoagulation therapy with healthcare providers to ensure appropriate treatment decisions.

4. Other Medications:

In addition to rate control, rhythm control, and anticoagulation therapy, individuals with AF may require other medications to manage coexisting medical conditions. These may include medications to control blood pressure, manage underlying heart diseases, control diabetes, or address specific comorbidities.

Medication therapy in AF should always be tailored to the individual patient, considering factors such as the type of AF (paroxysmal, persistent, or permanent), underlying health conditions, presence of structural heart disease, and individual treatment goals.

Regular follow-up appointments with healthcare providers are essential to monitor the efficacy and safety of medications, make necessary adjustments, and address any concerns or side effects.

It is important to note that medication therapy alone may not be sufficient for all individuals with AF, and other treatment options such as catheter ablation or surgical procedures may be considered in certain cases. The choice of treatment approach should be based on an individual's specific circumstances and discussed thoroughly with healthcare providers.

Remember, medication therapy in AF should always be prescribed and managed by qualified healthcare professionals to ensure optimal safety and efficacy.

Importance of Regular Exercise and Healthy Diet in Atrial Fibrillation

Regular exercise and a healthy diet are essential components of a comprehensive management plan for individuals with atrial fibrillation (AF). These lifestyle modifications play a crucial role in improving cardiovascular health, reducing AF symptoms, and enhancing overall well-being. Let's delve into the details of the importance of regular exercise and a healthy diet in AF:

1. Regular Exercise:
Engaging in regular physical activity offers numerous benefits for individuals with AF:

   a. Cardiovascular Fitness: Regular exercise improves cardiovascular fitness, strengthens the heart muscle, and enhances its ability to pump blood efficiently. This can lead to improved heart function and a reduced risk of AF-related complications.

b. Weight Management: Exercise helps maintain a healthy body weight or achieve weight loss when needed. Obesity and excess body weight are risk factors for AF, and weight reduction can significantly reduce the frequency and severity of AF episodes.

c. Stress Reduction: Physical activity has stress-reducing effects, promoting mental well-being and potentially reducing triggers for AF episodes. Managing stress through exercise, such as aerobic activities, yoga, or meditation, can contribute to better AF management.

d. Blood Pressure Control: Regular exercise helps lower blood pressure levels, reducing the strain on the heart and decreasing the risk of AF-related complications. It is particularly beneficial for individuals with hypertension, a common comorbidity with AF.

e. Improved Sleep: Exercise promotes better sleep quality, which can positively impact overall health and potentially reduce the risk of AF episodes triggered by sleep disturbances.

When incorporating exercise into an AF management plan, it is essential to consult with healthcare providers to determine the most appropriate types and intensity of exercise based on individual capabilities and any underlying health conditions.

2. Healthy Diet:

A well-balanced, heart-healthy diet is crucial for individuals with AF:

a. Nutrient-Rich Foods: A diet rich in fruits, vegetables, whole grains, lean proteins, and healthy fats provides essential nutrients that support heart health and overall well-being. These foods are typically low in saturated and trans fats, cholesterol, sodium, and added sugars.

b. Omega-3 Fatty Acids: Including sources of omega-3 fatty acids, such as fatty fish (salmon, mackerel, sardines), flaxseeds, and walnuts, in the diet may have protective effects on cardiovascular health and potentially reduce the risk of AF.

c. Limiting Sodium Intake: Reducing sodium (salt) intake is important for managing blood pressure and minimizing fluid retention. It involves avoiding processed and packaged foods high in sodium and using herbs, spices, and other flavor-enhancing techniques instead.

d. Fluid Intake: Adequate hydration is essential, but excessive fluid intake should be avoided, especially if fluid restriction is recommended by healthcare providers.

e. Alcohol and Caffeine: Limiting alcohol and caffeine intake is generally advised, as these substances can trigger AF episodes in some individuals.

A registered dietitian or healthcare provider can provide personalized dietary recommendations and guidance based on individual needs, preferences, and any specific dietary restrictions.

Regular exercise and a healthy diet should be pursued as long-term lifestyle changes rather than short-term interventions.

It is important to gradually increase exercise levels, stay consistent, and make dietary changes sustainable for optimal results. Additionally, it is crucial to work in collaboration with healthcare providers to ensure exercise and dietary recommendations are appropriate and aligned with individual needs and any other treatment strategies being utilized.

Remember, before making any significant changes to exercise or diet, consulting with healthcare providers is essential, particularly for individuals with specific medical conditions, mobility limitations, or other individual considerations.

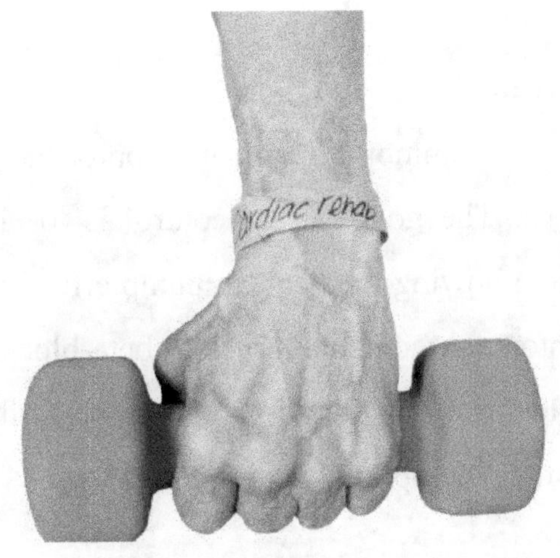

CHAPTER SEVEN

Treatment Options for Atrial Fibrillation

Atrial fibrillation (AF) is a complex condition that requires a comprehensive approach to management. The treatment options for AF aim to control symptoms, restore and maintain normal heart rhythm (sinus rhythm), prevent complications, and improve overall quality of life. The choice of treatment depends on several factors, including the type of AF, underlying health conditions, symptom severity, and individual patient preferences. Let's explore the various treatment options for atrial fibrillation:

1. Rate Control Strategy:

Rate control is a common treatment approach for individuals with AF. The goal of rate control is to slow down the heart rate, allowing the heart to pump effectively and reducing symptoms. Medications such as beta-blockers, calcium channel blockers, and digoxin are often prescribed to achieve and maintain an optimal heart rate.

2. Rhythm Control Strategy:

Rhythm control focuses on restoring and maintaining normal heart rhythm (sinus rhythm) in individuals with AF. This approach aims to eliminate or reduce AF episodes and associated symptoms. Antiarrhythmic medications, such as class I, class III, or sometimes class IC agents, may be prescribed to help restore and maintain sinus rhythm. In some cases, electrical cardioversion, a procedure where an electric shock is delivered to the heart, may be performed to restore normal heart rhythm.

3. Catheter Ablation:

Catheter ablation is a minimally invasive procedure used to treat AF by targeting and destroying the abnormal electrical pathways in the heart that cause AF. During the procedure, a catheter is guided to the heart, and energy sources (such as radiofrequency or cryotherapy) are used to create lesions or scar tissue to interrupt the abnormal electrical signals. Catheter ablation is considered for individuals with symptomatic AF who have not responded well to medication therapy or who prefer a more definitive treatment option.

4. Surgical Procedures:

In some cases, surgical interventions may be considered for AF management. Surgical procedures, such as maze procedures or minimally invasive techniques like thoracoscopic ablation, aim to create scar tissue in specific areas of the heart to block the abnormal electrical pathways causing AF. These procedures are often performed in conjunction with other cardiac surgeries, such as valve repair or coronary artery bypass grafting.

5. Anticoagulation Therapy:

Anticoagulation therapy is essential for individuals with AF to reduce the risk of blood clots, stroke, and systemic embolism. The decision to prescribe anticoagulants is based on an individual's risk factors for stroke, as assessed by scoring systems such as CHA2DS2-VASc. The two main types of anticoagulants used are vitamin K antagonists (such as warfarin) and direct oral anticoagulants (DOACs) like rivaroxaban, apixaban, dabigatran, and edoxaban. The choice of anticoagulant depends on individual factors such as age, renal function, bleeding risk, and concomitant medications.

6. Lifestyle Modifications:

A vital part of treating AF is altering one's lifestyle in addition to using medication therapies. These modifications include maintaining a healthy weight, adopting a heart-healthy diet, engaging in regular physical activity, managing stress levels, avoiding excessive alcohol and caffeine consumption, and quitting smoking. These lifestyle changes can contribute to better AF control and overall cardiovascular health.

It is important to note that the treatment approach for AF is highly individualized, and a combination of treatment modalities may be used depending on the specific needs of each patient. Treatment decisions should be made in consultation with healthcare providers, taking into account factors such as the type and duration of AF, symptom severity, risk of complications, and individual patient preferences.

Keeping up with follow-up consultations with medical professionals is crucial to monitor treatment efficacy, adjust medications if needed, and address any concerns or side effects. Treatment for AF is typically focused on long-term management and may require ongoing adjustments to optimize outcomes and ensure the best quality of life for individuals living with AF.

Pharmacological Treatment

Pharmacological treatment plays a significant role in the management of atrial fibrillation (AF). The primary goals of pharmacotherapy in AF are to control heart rate, maintain sinus rhythm, prevent thromboembolic events, and alleviate symptoms. The choice of medications depends on several factors, including the type of AF, underlying health conditions, patient characteristics, and individual preferences. Let's explore the different classes of medications commonly used in the pharmacological treatment of atrial fibrillation:

1. Antiarrhythmic Medications:

Antiarrhythmic drugs are used to restore and maintain normal sinus rhythm in individuals with AF. They work by suppressing abnormal electrical signals and preventing the initiation or recurrence of AF episodes. The choice of antiarrhythmic medication is influenced by the type of AF, presence of structural heart disease, renal and hepatic function, and potential drug interactions. Commonly prescribed antiarrhythmic agents include:

- **Class Ic Agents:** Drugs such as flecainide and propafenone are used to restore sinus rhythm and prevent AF recurrences in individuals without structural heart disease.

- **Class III Agents:** Medications like amiodarone, sotalol, and dofetilide are effective in maintaining sinus rhythm and reducing AF episodes. They are often prescribed for individuals with structural heart disease or those who have not responded to other antiarrhythmic agents.

2. Rate Control Medications:

Rate control medications are used to control the heart rate in individuals with AF. They work by slowing down the electrical impulses in the atria, allowing the ventricles to beat at a regular and controlled rate. Commonly prescribed rate control medications include:

- **Beta-Blockers:** Drugs such as metoprolol, atenolol, and carvedilol are frequently used to lower heart rate and control symptoms in AF. They are particularly beneficial for individuals with concomitant hypertension or heart failure.

- **Calcium Channel Blockers:** Medications like diltiazem and verapamil are used to slow down the heart rate and are often preferred for individuals with AF and coexisting conditions such as hypertension or coronary artery disease.

- **Digoxin:** Digoxin may be used in select cases to control heart rate in individuals with AF, particularly those with heart failure or when other rate control agents are contraindicated.

3. Anticoagulants:

Anticoagulants are essential for individuals with AF to prevent the formation of blood clots and reduce the risk of stroke and systemic embolism. Two main types of anticoagulants are commonly used:

- **Vitamin K Antagonists (VKAs):** Warfarin is a commonly prescribed VKA that requires regular monitoring of the international normalized ratio (INR) to ensure appropriate anticoagulation.

- **Direct Oral Anticoagulants (DOACs):** DOACs such as apixaban, dabigatran, edoxaban, and rivaroxaban offer more convenient dosing and do not require routine monitoring. They have demonstrated non-inferiority or superiority to warfarin in stroke prevention in AF.

4. Other Medications:

Additional medications may be prescribed to manage underlying conditions or risk factors associated with AF. These include:

- **Blood Pressure Medications:** Medications to control hypertension, such as angiotensin-converting enzyme inhibitors (ACE inhibitors), angiotensin II receptor blockers (ARBs), and diuretics, may be prescribed to manage blood pressure and reduce the risk of AF-related complications.

- **Thyroid Medications:** Individuals with AF and underlying thyroid dysfunction may require thyroid hormone replacement or antithyroid medications to achieve proper thyroid function, which can help stabilize heart rhythm.

It is important to note that medication therapy for AF should be individualized based on patient characteristics, comorbidities, and overall risk-benefit analysis. Regular follow-up appointments with healthcare providers are necessary to assess treatment efficacy, adjust medication dosages if needed, and monitor for any adverse effects or interactions. The ultimate goal of pharmacological treatment for AF is to optimize rhythm control, alleviate symptoms, reduce the risk of complications, and improve overall quality of life for individuals living with this condition.

Electrical Cardioversion and Ablation Procedures

Electrical cardioversion and ablation procedures are important interventions used in the management of atrial fibrillation (AF). These procedures aim to restore and maintain normal sinus rhythm, alleviate symptoms, and improve overall quality of life for individuals with AF. Let's explore the details of electrical cardioversion and ablation procedures in the context of atrial fibrillation:

1. Electrical Cardioversion:

Electrical cardioversion is a procedure that uses a controlled electric shock to restore normal sinus rhythm in individuals with AF. To ensure patient comfort, it is often carried out under sedation or general anesthesia. During the procedure, pads or paddles are placed on the chest, and an electrical shock is delivered to the heart, momentarily stopping its electrical activity. This "resets" the heart's electrical system, allowing the sinus node to regain control and establish normal rhythm.

Electrical cardioversion is commonly used for individuals with persistent or long-standing persistent AF who have failed to achieve sinus rhythm through pharmacological means alone. Prior to cardioversion, anticoagulation therapy is initiated for a period of time to reduce the risk of thromboembolic events associated with the restoration of sinus rhythm.

2. Catheter Ablation:

Catheter ablation is a minimally invasive procedure used to treat atrial fibrillation by targeting and eliminating the abnormal electrical pathways in the heart that cause AF. It is considered for individuals with symptomatic AF who have not responded well to medication therapy or those who prefer a more definitive treatment option.

During catheter ablation, thin, flexible catheters are inserted into the blood vessels and guided to the heart. These catheters deliver energy sources, such as radiofrequency or cryotherapy, to create lesions or scar tissue in specific areas of the heart. The scar tissue blocks the abnormal electrical signals that trigger AF, helping to restore normal sinus rhythm.

There are different types of catheter ablation procedures for AF, including pulmonary vein isolation (PVI), which targets the pulmonary veins that are often the sources of abnormal electrical impulses, and additional lesion sets that may be performed based on individual patient characteristics and the presence of other triggers or substrates.

Catheter ablation is a highly specialized procedure that requires expertise in electrophysiology. It is usually performed in a specialized cardiac electrophysiology laboratory by experienced healthcare professionals.

Both electrical cardioversion and catheter ablation have their own considerations and potential risks, and the decision to proceed with either procedure is based on individual patient factors, including the type and duration of AF, presence of structural heart disease, symptom severity, and response to prior treatments.

It is important to discuss these procedures with a cardiac electrophysiologist or healthcare provider specializing in the management of AF to determine the most appropriate treatment approach for each individual. These interventions can significantly improve symptoms, restore normal heart rhythm, and enhance the overall quality of life for individuals living with atrial fibrillation.

Surgical Interventions and Implantable Devices

Surgical interventions and implantable devices play a crucial role in the management of atrial fibrillation (AF). These interventions are typically considered for individuals with persistent or long-standing persistent AF, as well as those who have not responded well to other treatment options. Let's explore the details of surgical interventions and implantable devices used in the context of atrial fibrillation:

1. Maze Procedure:

The Maze procedure is a surgical intervention aimed at restoring normal sinus rhythm by creating a series of controlled scar lines or lesions in the atria. These scar lines redirect the electrical signals in the heart, allowing them to follow a more organized pathway and promoting the restoration of normal rhythm.

Traditional Maze surgery involves making several incisions in the atrial walls to create these scar lines. Nowadays, minimally invasive techniques, such as radiofrequency or cryotherapy, can also be used to create these lesions. The procedure can be performed as a stand-alone surgery or in combination with other cardiac surgeries, such as coronary artery bypass grafting or valve repair/replacement.

2. Pulmonary Vein Isolation (PVI) Surgery:

PVI surgery is a surgical procedure that aims to isolate the pulmonary veins from the left atrium to prevent the initiation and spread of abnormal electrical signals that cause atrial fibrillation.

During the procedure, the surgeon creates a circular or box-shaped lesion around the pulmonary veins to electrically isolate them from the rest of the atria.

PVI surgery can be performed using different techniques, including radiofrequency energy, cryotherapy, or even the use of specialized stapling devices. This procedure has shown promising results in maintaining sinus rhythm and reducing AF recurrence in select individuals.

3. Left Atrial Appendage Closure (LAAC):
The left atrial appendage (LAA) is a small pouch-like structure in the heart where blood can pool and potentially form blood clots. These blood clots can increase the risk of stroke in individuals with AF. Left atrial appendage closure (LAAC) procedures aim to seal off the LAA to reduce the risk of stroke.

LAAC can be achieved through surgical techniques, such as LAA excision or ligation, or through minimally invasive transcatheter approaches using specialized devices, such as occluders or plugs. These devices are placed inside the LAA to block its opening and prevent blood from entering.

4. Implantable Devices:

Implantable devices are also used in the management of atrial fibrillation, particularly for individuals at high risk of stroke or those with symptomatic AF who are not suitable candidates for anticoagulation therapy.

The two main types of implantable devices used in AF management are:

- Pacemakers: Pacemakers are commonly used in individuals with bradycardia (slow heart rate) or in those who require rate control in addition to rhythm control. Pacemakers can help maintain a regular heart rate and provide necessary electrical stimulation when the heart's natural pacemaker function is compromised.

- Implantable Cardioverter-Defibrillators (ICDs): ICDs are devices implanted in individuals at high risk of life-threatening ventricular arrhythmias, including those with AF. They continuously monitor the heart's rhythm and can deliver electrical shocks or pacing if a dangerous arrhythmia is detected, helping to restore normal rhythm.

The choice of surgical intervention or implantable device depends on various factors, including the individual's medical history, severity of AF, presence of structural heart disease, and response to prior treatments.

It is important to consult with a cardiac surgeon or an electrophysiologist to determine the most suitable surgical intervention or implantable device option for each individual. These interventions can significantly improve outcomes, restore normal heart rhythm, reduce the risk of complications, and enhance the overall quality of life for individuals living with atrial fibrillation.

Emerging Therapies and Future Directions

The field of atrial fibrillation (AF) management is continuously evolving, with ongoing research and advancements in treatment options. Emerging therapies and future directions in AF management aim to improve outcomes, enhance patient care, and address the challenges associated with this complex arrhythmia. Let's explore some of the promising emerging therapies and future directions in the management of atrial fibrillation:

1. Catheter-Based Therapies:

a. Hybrid Ablation: Hybrid ablation combines surgical and catheter-based ablation techniques to provide more comprehensive treatment for AF. It involves a minimally invasive surgical procedure, such as the Maze procedure, combined with subsequent catheter ablation to further target specific areas of the heart. This hybrid approach offers the potential for higher success rates in maintaining sinus rhythm.

b. Focal Impulse and Rotor Modulation (FIRM): FIRM is an innovative catheter-based therapy that targets localized electrical sources, known as rotors, in the atria. By identifying and ablating these rotors, FIRM aims to disrupt the AF triggers and maintain normal sinus rhythm.

c. Renal Denervation: Renal denervation is a procedure initially developed for treating hypertension. However, it has shown potential benefits in AF management as well. By targeting the sympathetic nervous system through radiofrequency ablation of the renal arteries, renal denervation aims to reduce the autonomic triggers associated with AF.

2. New Pharmacological Approaches:

a. Antiarrhythmic Drugs: Ongoing research focuses on the development of novel antiarrhythmic drugs that are more effective and safer in maintaining sinus rhythm and reducing AF burden. These medications target specific ion channels or receptors involved in the electrical conduction system of the heart, aiming to restore normal rhythm without significant adverse effects.

b. Novel Anticoagulants: Direct oral anticoagulants (DOACs) have revolutionized stroke prevention in AF by offering improved safety and convenience compared to traditional vitamin K antagonists. Ongoing research aims to further refine and personalize anticoagulation therapy by identifying biomarkers or genetic factors that may guide treatment decisions and optimize the balance between stroke prevention and bleeding risk.

3. Non-Invasive Therapies:

a. Transcutaneous Electrical Nerve Stimulation (TENS): TENS is a non-invasive technique that involves the application of low-intensity electrical currents to specific areas of the body. It has shown promise in reducing AF-related symptoms and improving quality of life. Ongoing studies are exploring its potential as an adjunctive therapy for AF management.

b. Neuromodulation: Neuromodulation techniques, such as vagus nerve stimulation, spinal cord stimulation, and transcranial magnetic stimulation, are being investigated for their potential in modulating autonomic nervous system activity and reducing AF burden. These non-invasive approaches aim to restore autonomic balance and improve heart rhythm.

4. Personalized Medicine and Precision Therapies:

The concept of personalized medicine is gaining momentum in AF management. Advances in genetic testing, imaging techniques, and electrophysiological mapping allow for a more individualized approach to treatment. Tailoring therapy based on an individual's genetic profile, structural heart abnormalities, or specific triggers may result in more effective and targeted interventions.

5. Artificial Intelligence and Digital Health:

Artificial intelligence (AI) and digital health technologies have the potential to revolutionize AF management.

AI algorithms can aid in the detection, prediction, and risk stratification of AF, allowing for early intervention and personalized treatment plans. Remote monitoring, wearable devices, and mobile applications enable continuous monitoring and engagement, facilitating proactive management and timely intervention.

It is important to note that emerging therapies and future directions in AF management are still under investigation, and their long-term efficacy and safety profiles are being evaluated. However, these advancements hold great promise for improving the outcomes and quality of life for individuals living with atrial fibrillation. As further research unfolds, these innovative approaches have the potential to shape the future landscape of AF management.

CHAPTER EIGHT

Living with Atrial Fibrillation

Atrial fibrillation (AF) is a chronic condition that requires long-term management. While it can present challenges, with proper care and lifestyle adjustments, individuals with AF can lead fulfilling lives. Here is a professional and detailed overview of living with atrial fibrillation:

1. Education and Understanding:

Understanding the nature of AF, its symptoms, and its management is crucial for individuals with the condition. Educate yourself about AF, its causes, risk factors, treatment options, and potential complications. With this information, you are more equipped to take an active role in your treatment and make wise choices.

2. Medication Adherence:

Strict adherence to prescribed medications is essential for managing AF. Medications may include antiarrhythmic drugs, anticoagulants, beta-blockers, or other medications to control heart rate and rhythm.

Follow your healthcare provider's instructions regarding dosage, timing, and potential interactions with other medications.

3. Lifestyle Modifications:

Lifestyle modifications play a significant role in managing AF and reducing its impact on your daily life. Consider the following:

a. Healthy Diet: Adopt a heart-healthy diet that includes fruits, vegetables, whole grains, lean proteins, and limited saturated fats, cholesterol, and sodium. This helps maintain a healthy weight, manage blood pressure, and reduce the risk of other cardiovascular conditions.

b. Regular Exercise: Engage in regular physical activity based on your healthcare provider's recommendations. Aim for at least 150 minutes of moderate-intensity aerobic exercise per week, such as brisk walking, cycling, swimming, or other activities that you enjoy. Prior to beginning any fitness regimen, speak with your healthcare provider.

c. Stress Management: Develop strategies to manage stress, as stress can trigger or exacerbate AF episodes. Practice relaxation techniques, such as deep breathing, meditation, yoga, or engaging in activities that promote relaxation and well-being.

d. Avoid Triggers: Identify and avoid factors that may trigger AF episodes or worsen symptoms. Common triggers include excessive alcohol consumption, caffeine, smoking, certain medications, and illicit drugs. Keep a record of potential triggers and discuss them with your healthcare provider.

4. Regular Medical Follow-up:

Regular medical follow-up is crucial to monitor your AF and adjust your treatment plan as needed. Attend scheduled appointments with your healthcare provider and undergo recommended tests, such as electrocardiograms, echocardiograms, or blood tests, to assess your heart rhythm, function, and overall health.

5. Stroke Prevention:

Stroke prevention is a critical aspect of AF management due to the increased risk of blood clots forming in the atria. Your healthcare provider may prescribe anticoagulant medications to reduce this risk. It is essential to take these medications as directed and undergo regular monitoring to ensure their effectiveness.

6. Support System:

Building a strong support system can be beneficial when living with AF. Share your experiences and concerns with loved ones, join support groups, or consider seeking professional counseling to help you cope with the emotional and psychological impact of the condition.

7. Stay Informed:

Stay up to date with the latest developments in AF management. Attend educational seminars, read reputable sources, and engage with your healthcare provider to stay informed about advancements in treatment options, emerging therapies, and self-care strategies.

Remember, each individual's experience with AF is unique, and it may take time to find the right combination of treatments and lifestyle adjustments that work for you. Work closely with your healthcare team to develop a personalized management plan that addresses your specific needs and goals. With proper care and support, you can lead a fulfilling life while effectively managing atrial fibrillation.

Coping Strategies and Emotional Support

Coping with atrial fibrillation (AF) involves not only managing the physical aspects of the condition but also addressing the emotional and psychological impact it can have on individuals. Here are some professional and detailed coping strategies and emotional support options for individuals with AF:

1. Education and Self-Management:

Educate yourself about AF and its management. Understanding the condition can help alleviate anxiety and empower you to actively participate in your care. Learn about lifestyle modifications, medications, treatment options, and self-monitoring techniques to better manage your condition.

2. Supportive Healthcare Team:

Build a strong partnership with your healthcare team, including your cardiologist, electrophysiologist, nurses, and other healthcare professionals. Regular communication and open discussions about your concerns, questions, and treatment plan can provide reassurance and help you feel supported.

3. Emotional Expression and Communication:

Express your feelings and emotions regarding AF with trusted friends, family members, or support groups. Sharing your experiences can provide a sense of validation, reduce feelings of isolation, and offer opportunities for emotional support.

Effective communication with your loved ones can also help them understand your condition and provide the support you need.

4. Stress Management Techniques:

Stress is a known trigger for AF episodes. Incorporate stress management techniques into your daily routine to promote relaxation and emotional well-being. Consider activities such as deep breathing exercises, meditation, mindfulness, yoga, or engaging in hobbies and activities that bring you joy and peace.

5. Emotional Support Groups:

Joining support groups or online communities specific to AF can provide a platform to connect with others who share similar experiences. These groups offer opportunities to discuss concerns, exchange coping strategies, and gain emotional support from individuals who understand the challenges associated with living with AF.

6. Psychological Counseling:

Consider seeking professional counseling or therapy to address any psychological or emotional challenges you may be facing. A mental health professional experienced in working with individuals with chronic conditions can provide guidance, help you develop coping mechanisms, and assist in navigating the emotional impact of AF.

7. Healthy Lifestyle:

To support your general well-being, maintain a healthy lifestyle. Engage in regular exercise, follow a balanced diet, get adequate sleep, and avoid excessive alcohol consumption and smoking. A healthy lifestyle can positively impact both your physical and emotional health, potentially reducing the frequency and severity of AF episodes.

8. Mind-Body Techniques:

Explore mind-body techniques such as relaxation exercises, biofeedback, acupuncture, or massage therapy.

These complementary approaches can promote relaxation, reduce stress, and contribute to a sense of overall well-being.

9. Personal Well-Being:

Concentrate on self-care and pursuits that make you happy and content. Engage in hobbies, pursue interests, practice self-compassion, and prioritize self-care routines. Nurturing your personal well-being can help you maintain a positive outlook and improve your overall quality of life.

10. Regular Follow-up:

Attend regular follow-up appointments with your healthcare provider to monitor your AF and address any concerns or changes in your condition. Regular check-ins can provide reassurance, ensure appropriate management, and give you an opportunity to discuss any emotional or psychological aspects related to AF.

Remember, it is normal to experience a range of emotions when living with a chronic condition like AF.

Taking proactive steps to address the emotional impact, seeking support, and developing coping strategies can help you navigate the challenges and maintain a positive outlook.

Patient Education and Self-Care Practices

Patient education and self-care practices are essential components of managing atrial fibrillation (AF) effectively. Empowering individuals with knowledge about their condition and equipping them with self-care strategies can improve their quality of life and promote better management of AF. Here is a professional and detailed overview of patient education and self-care practices for individuals with AF:

1. Understanding Atrial Fibrillation:

Educate yourself about AF, its causes, symptoms, treatment options, and potential complications. Understand the underlying mechanisms of AF, how it affects your heart rhythm, and the associated cardiovascular risks.

This knowledge will enable you to make informed decisions and actively participate in your care.

2. Medication Adherence:

As instructed by your healthcare professional, follow the medication schedule you have been prescribed. Take medications on time, at the recommended dosage, and be aware of any potential side effects or interactions with other medications. If you have concerns or questions about your medications, discuss them with your healthcare team.

3. Lifestyle Modifications:

Adopting a healthy lifestyle can significantly impact the management of AF. Consider the following self-care practices:

a. Healthy Diet: Follow a balanced diet that includes fruits, vegetables, whole grains, lean proteins, and limited saturated fats, cholesterol, and sodium. A heart-healthy diet can help maintain a healthy weight, manage blood pressure, and support overall cardiovascular health.

b. Regular Exercise: Engage in regular physical activity, as recommended by your healthcare provider. Strive for 150 minutes or more per week of aerobic activity at a moderate level. Activities such as walking, cycling, swimming, or dancing can help improve cardiovascular fitness and overall well-being. Prior to beginning an exercise regimen, speak with your healthcare professional.

c. Stress Management: Develop stress management techniques to minimize the impact of stress on your AF. Use relaxation techniques like yoga, meditation, deep breathing, or mindfulness. Engage in activities that promote relaxation and emotional well-being, such as spending time in nature, listening to calming music, or pursuing hobbies you enjoy.

d. Alcohol and Caffeine Intake: Limit your alcohol consumption, as excessive alcohol can trigger AF episodes. Monitor your caffeine intake and consider reducing it if you notice a correlation between caffeine and AF symptoms.

e. Smoking Cessation: If you smoke, quitting is crucial for managing AF. Smoking can exacerbate the condition and increase the risk of complications. Seek support from healthcare professionals, support groups, or smoking cessation programs to help you quit.

4. Stroke Prevention:

Work with your healthcare provider to assess your risk of stroke and implement appropriate preventive measures. This may include anticoagulant medications, such as warfarin or direct oral anticoagulants (DOACs), to reduce the risk of blood clots. Adhere to your prescribed anticoagulation therapy and undergo regular monitoring as recommended.

5. Self-Monitoring:

Engage in self-monitoring practices to track your AF symptoms, heart rate, and rhythm. This may involve regularly checking your pulse, using a personal ECG device, or using mobile applications that allow you to record and share data with your healthcare provider.

Self-monitoring helps you stay informed about your condition and detect any changes or irregularities.

6. Regular Medical Follow-up:

Attend scheduled follow-up appointments with your healthcare provider to assess the progress of your AF management. These visits may include electrocardiograms, echocardiograms, or blood tests to monitor your heart rhythm, evaluate your heart function, and ensure your treatment plan remains optimal.

7. Patient Resources and Support:

Take advantage of patient resources and support services available to you. Access reputable online sources, patient education materials, and support groups dedicated to AF. These resources can provide valuable information, emotional support, and opportunities to connect with individuals who share similar experiences.

By actively engaging in patient education and implementing self-care practices, you can play an active role in managing your AF.

Working in partnership with your healthcare team, adopting a healthy lifestyle, and staying informed about your condition will empower you to lead a fulfilling life while effectively managing AF.

Monitoring and Follow-up Care

Monitoring and follow-up care play a crucial role in the effective management of atrial fibrillation (AF). Regular monitoring allows healthcare providers to assess the progress of your treatment, make necessary adjustments, and identify any potential complications. Here is a professional and detailed overview of monitoring and follow-up care for individuals with AF:

1. Frequency of Follow-up Visits:

Your healthcare provider will determine the frequency of your follow-up visits based on the severity of your AF, treatment plan, and individual needs. Typically, follow-up visits occur every three to six months, but this may vary. Adhering to the recommended schedule ensures ongoing evaluation of your condition and timely intervention if needed.

2. Physical Examination:

During each follow-up visit, your healthcare provider will conduct a thorough physical examination. This may include measuring your blood pressure, checking your heart rate and rhythm, and assessing any signs or symptoms of AF or associated complications. Physical examinations help evaluate your overall cardiovascular health and monitor the progression of AF.

3. Electrocardiogram (ECG):

Regular ECGs are essential for monitoring your heart's electrical activity and detecting any changes in rhythm. Your healthcare provider may perform an ECG during each follow-up visit or as needed. The results provide valuable information about the duration and severity of AF episodes, allowing for adjustments to your treatment plan.

4. Holter Monitoring and Event Recorders:

In some cases, your healthcare provider may recommend additional monitoring tools such as Holter monitoring or event recorders.

Holter monitoring includes wearing a portable device that continually records the electrical activity of your heart for 24 to 48 hours or more. Event recorders are small devices that you activate when you experience symptoms, allowing for immediate recording of your heart rhythm. These monitoring methods help capture intermittent or infrequent AF episodes and provide valuable data for treatment optimization.

5. Echocardiography:

Echocardiography is a non-invasive imaging technique that uses ultrasound waves to evaluate the structure and function of your heart. It provides detailed information about the size of your heart chambers, the strength of your heart muscle, and the presence of any structural abnormalities. Echocardiograms are performed periodically to assess your heart's health and monitor any changes related to AF or its complications.

6. Blood Tests:

Blood tests are commonly performed during follow-up visits to monitor specific markers associated with AF and its treatment. These may include tests to assess thyroid function, electrolyte levels, kidney function, and the effectiveness of anticoagulation therapy. Blood tests provide valuable information about your overall health and help guide treatment decisions.

7. Assessment of Anticoagulation Therapy:

If you are prescribed anticoagulant medications to reduce the risk of stroke, your healthcare provider will monitor the effectiveness of the therapy through regular blood tests, such as the international normalized ratio (INR) for warfarin or specific tests for direct oral anticoagulants (DOACs). Adjustments to your medication dosage may be made to maintain the appropriate anticoagulation level.

8. Lifestyle and Medication Review:

During follow-up visits, your healthcare provider will assess your adherence to lifestyle modifications and medication regimen.

They will review your diet, exercise routine, alcohol and caffeine consumption, smoking habits, and stress management practices. Any necessary adjustments or recommendations will be provided to optimize your lifestyle and medication choices.

9. Ongoing Education and Counseling:

Follow-up visits provide an opportunity for ongoing patient education and counseling. Your healthcare provider will address any questions or concerns you may have, provide updates on advancements in AF management, and offer guidance on self-care practices. Education and counseling empower you to make informed decisions and actively participate in the management of your AF.

10. Care Coordination:

Follow-up visits also allow for care coordination with other healthcare professionals involved in your AF management, such as cardiologists, electrophysiologists, and specialized nurses. Collaboration among healthcare providers ensures comprehensive care, shared expertise, and effective communication regarding your treatment plan.

Regular monitoring and follow-up care are essential for optimizing the management of AF, ensuring the effectiveness of your treatment, and addressing any emerging concerns promptly. By actively participating in these processes, you can work closely with your healthcare team to achieve better outcomes and improve your overall quality of life.

Role of Caregivers and Support Networks

Caregivers and support networks play a crucial role in the management and well-being of individuals with atrial fibrillation (AF). The physical and emotional support provided by caregivers, family members, and friends can significantly impact the overall experience of living with AF. Here is a professional and detailed overview of the role of caregivers and support networks in AF:

1. Understanding AF and its Impact:

Caregivers and support networks should make an effort to understand AF, its causes, symptoms, and treatment options.

By gaining knowledge about the condition, they can better support and advocate for the individual with AF. Understanding the potential impact of AF on daily life, including limitations, risks, and challenges, allows caregivers to provide appropriate assistance and guidance.

2. Emotional Support:

Living with AF can be emotionally challenging for individuals. Caregivers and support networks can provide emotional support by being empathetic, understanding, and actively listening. Offering a safe space for individuals to express their feelings, concerns, and frustrations can be immensely valuable. Encouraging open communication and providing reassurance can help alleviate anxiety and stress associated with AF.

3. Assisting with Medication Management:

Caregivers can play a vital role in medication management for individuals with AF. This includes ensuring that medications are taken as prescribed, monitoring any side effects, and assisting with organizing and refilling prescriptions.

Caregivers can also help individuals keep track of their medication schedule and ensure they attend medical appointments and follow-up visits.

4. Encouraging Lifestyle Modifications:

Caregivers and support networks can help individuals with AF adopt and maintain healthy lifestyle modifications. This includes encouraging regular physical activity, promoting a nutritious diet, and supporting efforts to quit smoking and reduce alcohol consumption. By actively participating in these lifestyle changes, caregivers can create a supportive environment that fosters overall cardiovascular health.

5. Providing Practical Support:

Caregivers can offer practical assistance in various aspects of daily life. This may involve helping with household chores, transportation to medical appointments, and managing logistics related to AF management, such as scheduling tests or procedures. Offering practical support allows individuals with AF to focus on their health and well-being without feeling overwhelmed by everyday tasks.

6. Educating and Empowering:

Caregivers can educate themselves about AF and its management, enabling them to actively participate in decision-making processes alongside the individual with AF and the healthcare team. By staying informed about the latest advancements, treatment options, and self-care practices, caregivers can provide valuable input and help individuals make informed choices.

7. Supporting Self-Care Practices:

Caregivers can encourage and support self-care practices in individuals with AF. This includes promoting stress management techniques, assisting with meal planning and preparation of heart-healthy meals, and engaging in activities that promote relaxation and emotional well-being. By actively participating in self-care practices, caregivers can positively influence the overall health and well-being of individuals with AF.

8. Facilitating Communication with Healthcare Providers:

Caregivers can serve as advocates for individuals with AF during medical appointments and interactions with healthcare providers. They can help ensure that important questions are asked, concerns are addressed, and treatment plans are fully understood. Caregivers can also help individuals communicate their symptoms, experiences, and treatment response accurately to healthcare providers.

9. Encouraging Participation in Support Groups:

Caregivers can help individuals connect with support groups or online communities specifically focused on AF. These platforms provide opportunities for individuals to share experiences, exchange information, and seek emotional support from others who understand the challenges of living with AF. Caregivers can facilitate participation in these support networks, fostering a sense of belonging and reducing feelings of isolation.

10. Promoting Overall Well-being:

Caregivers can promote the overall well-being of individuals with AF by encouraging a positive mindset, engaging in enjoyable activities together, and supporting hobbies and interests. By fostering a nurturing and supportive environment, caregivers contribute to the individual's overall quality of life and mental well-being.

The role of caregivers and support networks in the management of AF is invaluable. Their support, understanding, and assistance can significantly enhance the physical, emotional, and social well-being of individuals living with AF. By working collaboratively with healthcare providers and individuals with AF, caregivers can play an essential part in optimizing AF management and improving the overall quality of life for everyone involved.

CONCLUSION

Atrial fibrillation (AF) is a complex cardiac condition that requires comprehensive understanding, timely diagnosis, and appropriate management. Throughout this guide, we have explored various aspects of AF, including its definition, causes, risk factors, symptoms, diagnosis, treatment options, and the impact it has on the lives of individuals.

AF is a prevalent arrhythmia that can lead to significant complications, such as stroke, heart failure, and impaired quality of life. However, with early detection, proper medical intervention, and lifestyle modifications, the prognosis for individuals with AF can be improved, and the risk of complications can be reduced.

Understanding the underlying causes of AF, including medical conditions, lifestyle factors, and environmental influences, is crucial in implementing effective preventive measures.

Lifestyle modifications, such as maintaining a healthy diet, engaging in regular exercise, managing stress, and avoiding excessive alcohol and tobacco use, play a vital role in reducing the risk of AF and its associated complications.

Timely diagnosis and ongoing monitoring of AF are essential for optimizing treatment strategies and managing the condition effectively. Diagnostic tools and tests, including electrocardiograms (ECGs), echocardiography, and blood tests, provide valuable insights into the severity and progression of AF, helping healthcare providers tailor individualized treatment plans.

Treatment options for AF include pharmacological interventions, electrical cardioversion, ablation procedures, surgical interventions, and implantable devices. The selection of treatment depends on factors such as the underlying cause, symptom severity, and individual patient characteristics. Anticoagulation therapy is crucial in reducing the risk of stroke and thromboembolism in individuals with AF, and adherence to medication regimens is paramount.

Living with AF requires a multidimensional approach that encompasses not only medical management but also emotional support, lifestyle modifications, self-care practices, and the involvement of caregivers and support networks. Through education, communication, and collaboration, individuals with AF can lead fulfilling lives while effectively managing their condition.

In conclusion, atrial fibrillation is a complex cardiac condition that necessitates a comprehensive approach to diagnosis, treatment, and ongoing management. By understanding the causes, recognizing symptoms, and implementing preventive measures, individuals with AF can take proactive steps towards maintaining a healthy heart and minimizing the risk of complications. With the support of healthcare providers, caregivers, and a strong network of emotional and practical support, individuals with AF can lead fulfilling lives, promoting their overall well-being and enhancing their quality of life.

Summary of Key Points for Atrial Fibrillation

1. Atrial fibrillation (AF) is a common cardiac arrhythmia characterized by irregular and rapid heartbeats originating from the atria of the heart.

2. AF can have various causes, including underlying medical conditions, lifestyle factors, and environmental influences. Understanding the causes is crucial for implementing preventive measures.

3. Recognizing the symptoms of AF is important for early detection and prompt medical intervention. Symptoms may include palpitations, shortness of breath, fatigue, dizziness, and chest discomfort.

4. Proper diagnosis of AF involves the use of diagnostic tools and tests such as electrocardiograms (ECGs), echocardiography, blood tests, Holter monitoring, and event recorders.

5. AF is associated with an increased risk of complications, including stroke, heart failure, and cardiac remodeling. Timely diagnosis, monitoring, and treatment are essential for minimizing these risks.

6. Treatment options for AF include lifestyle modifications, medication management, electrical cardioversion, catheter ablation, surgical interventions, and implantable devices. The choice of treatment depends on the individual's specific condition and needs.

7. Anticoagulation therapy is crucial for individuals with AF to reduce the risk of stroke and thromboembolism. It is important to adhere to prescribed medications and regular monitoring.

8. Living with AF requires a multidimensional approach, including self-care practices, lifestyle modifications, emotional support, and involvement of caregivers and support networks.

9. Regular follow-up visits and monitoring are important for optimizing AF management, adjusting treatment plans, and addressing any emerging concerns promptly.

10. Individualized patient education is essential for empowering individuals with AF to actively participate in their own care and make informed decisions regarding their treatment and lifestyle choices.

In conclusion, atrial fibrillation is a complex cardiac condition that requires a comprehensive approach to diagnosis, treatment, and ongoing management. By understanding the causes, recognizing symptoms, and implementing preventive measures, individuals with AF can reduce the risk of complications and improve their quality of life. With proper medical care, lifestyle modifications, and support from healthcare providers, caregivers, and support networks, individuals with AF can effectively manage their condition and lead fulfilling lives.

Empowering Individuals with Knowledge and Resources

Empowering individuals with atrial fibrillation (AF) with knowledge and resources is essential for their active involvement in managing their condition and making informed decisions about their health. By providing comprehensive education and access to relevant resources, healthcare professionals can empower individuals with AF to take control of their health and improve their overall well-being. Here is a professional, captivating, and detailed overview of how to empower individuals with AF through knowledge and resources:

1. Education on AF:

Providing individuals with AF with a clear understanding of their condition is crucial. Educate them about the causes, symptoms, and potential complications of AF. Explain how AF affects the heart's rhythm and the associated risks. Help individuals grasp the importance of timely diagnosis, monitoring, and adherence to treatment.

2. Treatment Options:

Explain the various treatment options available for AF, including lifestyle modifications, medications, procedures, and surgical interventions. Discuss the benefits, risks, and expected outcomes of each option, enabling individuals to make informed decisions in consultation with their healthcare team.

3. Self-Care Practices:

Educate individuals on self-care practices that can complement medical treatment. This includes stress management techniques, regular exercise, a heart-healthy diet, adequate sleep, and avoiding triggers such as excessive alcohol or caffeine. Provide practical tips and resources to help individuals incorporate these practices into their daily lives.

4. Medication Understanding:

Ensure that individuals fully understand their prescribed medications, including their purpose, dosage, potential side effects, and interactions with other medications.

Encourage open communication about any concerns or challenges they may face in adhering to their medication regimen.

5. Lifestyle Modifications:

Empower individuals with AF to make positive lifestyle changes that support their heart health. Educate them on the benefits of maintaining a healthy weight, quitting smoking, limiting alcohol consumption, and managing underlying health conditions such as high blood pressure and diabetes. Provide resources and support to facilitate these changes.

6. Risk Management:

Help individuals understand the importance of managing their overall cardiovascular risk factors. Educate them about the link between AF and other conditions such as hypertension, diabetes, and obesity. Encourage regular check-ups, blood pressure monitoring, and cholesterol management to reduce the risk of complications.

7. Support Networks:

Connect individuals with AF to support networks and patient advocacy organizations. These resources provide a platform for sharing experiences, gathering information, and finding emotional support from others who understand the challenges of living with AF. Offer guidance on reputable online forums, local support groups, and educational events.

8. Decision-Making and Shared Decision-Making:

Encourage individuals to actively participate in their healthcare decisions. Facilitate open and honest conversations with healthcare providers, allowing individuals to voice their concerns, ask questions, and share their treatment preferences. Shared decision-making empowers individuals and helps ensure that treatment plans align with their goals and values.

9. Clear Communication:

Foster a culture of clear and effective communication between individuals with AF, their healthcare providers, and caregivers.

Provide resources such as written materials, educational videos, and interactive tools that explain medical terminology and concepts in a user-friendly manner.

10. Ongoing Support:

Ensure that individuals have access to ongoing support and follow-up care. Schedule regular check-ins to address any questions or concerns and monitor treatment progress. Provide contact information for healthcare providers and encourage individuals to reach out whenever needed.

Empowering individuals with AF with knowledge and resources empowers them to actively participate in their own care, make informed decisions, and adopt healthy lifestyle practices. By working collaboratively with healthcare providers and having access to relevant educational materials and support networks, individuals with AF can effectively manage their condition, reduce complications, and improve their overall quality of life.

APPENDICES

Appendix I: Glossary of Terms

- This appendix provides a comprehensive list of medical terms and acronyms commonly associated with atrial fibrillation (AF) for easy reference and understanding.

Appendix A: Medication Guide

- This appendix includes a detailed guide on the medications commonly used for the treatment of AF. It provides information on dosage, common side effects, and precautions for each medication.

Appendix B: Sample Meal Plan

- A sample meal plan is included in this appendix, providing individuals with AF a practical guide for maintaining a heart-healthy diet. It includes nutritious meal options, portion sizes, and dietary recommendations.

Appendix C: Exercise Guide

- This appendix offers a detailed exercise guide specifically tailored for individuals with AF. It includes safe and effective exercises that promote cardiovascular health and provide guidelines on frequency, intensity, and duration of exercise.

Appendix D: Resource List

- The resource list compiles a collection of credible sources, websites, books, and other references related to AF. It provides individuals with AF a wealth of additional information and support resources they can explore.

Appendix E: Symptom Tracker

- This appendix includes a printable symptom tracker that individuals can use to monitor and record their AF symptoms. It helps in tracking the frequency, duration, and severity of symptoms, aiding in discussions with healthcare providers.

Appendix F: Contacts and Emergency Information

- This appendix contains important contact information for healthcare providers, emergency services, and support organizations. It serves as a quick reference in case of emergencies or the need for immediate medical assistance.

Appendix G: Notes and Journal

- Individuals can use this appendix to keep a personal journal or make notes related to their AF journey. It allows them to document their experiences, concerns, questions, and progress, facilitating better communication with healthcare providers.

Appendix II: Frequently Asked Questions (FAQs)

- This appendix addresses common questions and concerns individuals may have about AF.

It provides detailed answers to help clarify doubts and misconceptions, promoting a better understanding of the condition.

Note: The appendices are included to provide additional resources, tools, and information to supplement the main content of the guide. Individuals can refer to these appendices as needed for further guidance and support throughout their journey with AF.

Frequently Asked Questions (FAQs)

1. What is atrial fibrillation (AF)?

- Atrial fibrillation is a common heart rhythm disorder characterized by irregular and often rapid electrical impulses in the atria, the upper chambers of the heart. This can lead to an irregular heartbeat and other symptoms.

2. What are the common symptoms of AF?

- Common symptoms of AF include palpitations (racing, pounding, or irregular heartbeat), shortness of breath, fatigue, dizziness, chest discomfort, and fainting.

However, some individuals with AF may not experience any noticeable symptoms.

3. What causes atrial fibrillation?

- The causes of AF can vary, but common factors include underlying heart conditions such as hypertension, coronary artery disease, heart valve problems, and structural heart defects. Other factors include aging, thyroid disorders, excessive alcohol consumption, obesity, and certain medications or stimulants.

4. How is atrial fibrillation diagnosed?

- Diagnosis of AF involves a thorough medical history review, physical examination, and various tests such as electrocardiogram (ECG), echocardiogram, Holter monitoring, and blood tests. These tests help determine the presence of AF, assess its severity, and identify any underlying causes or associated complications.

5. What are the treatment options for atrial fibrillation?

- Treatment options for AF aim to control heart rate, restore normal heart rhythm, and prevent complications.

  They may include medications (such as antiarrhythmics and anticoagulants), electrical cardioversion, catheter ablation, surgical interventions, and lifestyle modifications.

6. How can lifestyle modifications help manage atrial fibrillation?

- Lifestyle modifications play a crucial role in managing AF. This includes adopting a heart-healthy diet, engaging in regular physical activity, managing stress, quitting smoking, limiting alcohol and caffeine intake, and maintaining a healthy weight. These lifestyle changes can help reduce symptoms, improve overall cardiovascular health, and enhance the effectiveness of medical treatments.

7. What are the potential complications of atrial fibrillation?

- AF can lead to complications such as an increased risk of stroke and blood clots, heart failure, cardiac remodeling, and other heart-related issues. Timely diagnosis, appropriate treatment, and management of underlying health conditions are important to minimize these risks.

8. Can atrial fibrillation be cured?

- While AF is a chronic condition, it can be effectively managed and controlled with the right treatment approach. In some cases, treatments such as catheter ablation or surgical interventions may restore normal heart rhythm, providing long-term relief. However, ongoing monitoring and management are generally necessary.

9. Can atrial fibrillation be prevented?

- While some risk factors for AF, such as age and family history, cannot be changed, certain lifestyle modifications and risk factor management can help reduce the risk of developing AF. This includes maintaining a healthy lifestyle, managing underlying health conditions, and avoiding triggers such as excessive alcohol and tobacco use.

10. How important is regular follow-up care for individuals with atrial fibrillation?

- Regular follow-up care is crucial for individuals with AF to monitor their condition, adjust treatment plans if needed, and address any emerging concerns. This allows healthcare providers to assess the effectiveness of treatment, monitor for complications, and make necessary adjustments to optimize the individual's heart health and overall well-being.

Note: These FAQs provide general information and answers to commonly asked questions about atrial fibrillation. It is important to consult with a healthcare professional for personalized advice and guidance regarding individual cases of AF.

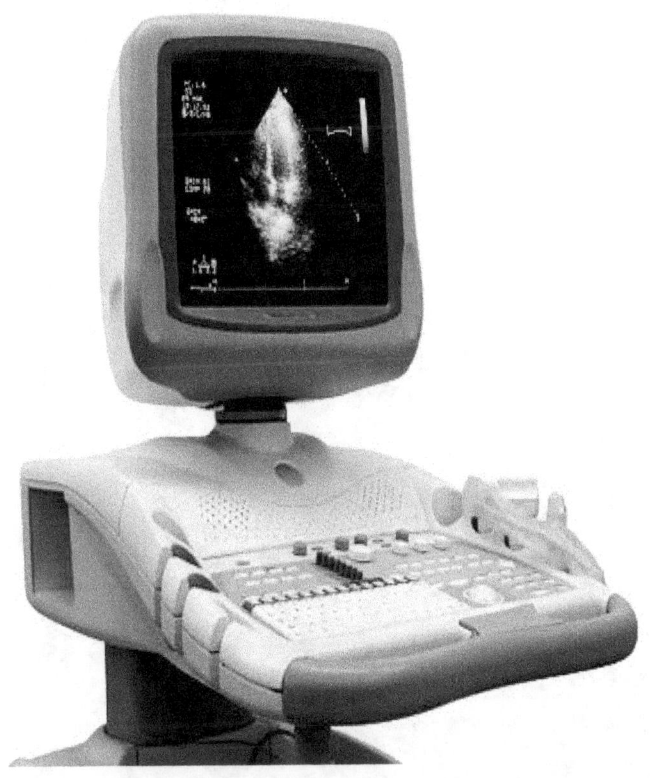